Mastering Clinical Judgment

50 Practical NGN-Ready Scenarios for Nursing Students

Irvin Eliane Harrison

Mastering Clinical Judgment:50 Practical NGN-Ready Scenarios for Nursing Students

inaccuracies in clinical content, or changes in professional standards or practice guidelines that occur after publication.

All patient names, healthcare provider names, and institutional names used in this publication are entirely fictional. Any resemblance to actual persons, living or deceased, or to actual healthcare institutions is purely coincidental and unintentional. No real patient information, protected health information (PHI), or actual clinical cases have been used in the development of this educational material. References to established nursing theories, clinical judgment models, and educational frameworks are used for educational purposes with proper attribution where applicable.

References to Next Generation NCLEX (NGN) question formats and the National Council of State Boards of Nursing (NCSBN) Clinical Judgment Measurement Model are used for educational context. This publication is not affiliated with, endorsed by, or officially connected to the NCSBN or the NCLEX examination program. This book is not intended to replace official NCLEX preparation materials or guarantee success on the NCLEX examination.

The author, Irvin Eliane Harrison, and the publisher shall not be liable for any direct, indirect, incidental, special, consequential, or punitive damages arising out of the use of or inability to use the information contained in this publication, even if advised of the possibility of such damages. Healthcare knowledge and practice standards evolve continuously. While every effort has been made to ensure accuracy at the time of publication, readers are encouraged to consult current literature and evidence-based resources, verify information with authoritative sources, and report any errors or concerns to the publisher for consideration in future editions.

ISBN: 978-1-7642235-5-3

Isohan Publishing

Table of Contents

Chapter 1: Introduction to Clinical Judgment in Nursing

Clinical judgment represents the cornerstone of safe, effective nursing practice. Each decision you make at the bedside carries weight—not just in terms of patient outcomes, but in your development as a professional nurse. The nursing profession has recognized this reality and responded with significant changes to how we prepare and assess future nurses.

The Evolution of Clinical Judgment Assessment

The transformation from traditional NCLEX to the Next Generation NCLEX (NGN) in April 2023 marks a watershed moment in nursing education. This shift didn't happen overnight. Years of research demonstrated that newly licensed nurses struggled with clinical decision-making despite passing traditional examinations (1). The National Council of State Boards of Nursing (NCSBN) recognized that testing factual recall and basic application wasn't enough—nurses needed assessment methods that truly measured their ability to think through complex patient situations.

Consider Sarah, a new graduate who excelled in nursing school. She memorized every drug dosage, aced her pathophysiology exams, and passed the traditional NCLEX on her first attempt. Yet during her first month on a medical-surgical unit, she froze when her patient developed chest pain. She knew the textbook symptoms of myocardial infarction, but connecting those symptoms to her specific patient, prioritizing her actions, and adapting when the initial interventions didn't provide expected results—these skills required a different kind of thinking altogether.

The evidence supporting this change is compelling. Studies showed that 23% of newly licensed nurses experienced "transition shock," feeling unprepared for the clinical reasoning demands of practice (2). Hospital administrators reported that new graduates required longer orientation periods and more intensive preceptorship than in previous decades. Patient safety data revealed that clinical judgment errors contributed to significant adverse events, particularly among novice nurses (3).

The NGN addresses these concerns by incorporating the Clinical Judgment Measurement Model (CJMM), which tests your ability to recognize relevant patient data, analyze its significance, prioritize your responses, plan interventions, implement care, and evaluate outcomes. This mirrors what you actually do in clinical practice—not just what you know, but how you think.

Book Structure and Learning Approach

This book operates on a progressive complexity framework designed to mirror your natural learning progression. Think of it as scaffolding for your clinical judgment development. Just as you wouldn't expect to perform complex procedures without first mastering basic skills, you shouldn't expect to handle multi-system patient crises without first developing judgment skills with straightforward scenarios.

The 50 scenarios in this book follow three distinct levels:

Beginner scenarios focus on single-system problems with clear protocols. These scenarios help you practice recognizing and analyzing cues when the clinical picture is relatively straightforward. You'll work through situations like managing stable hypertension or providing post-operative care, where established guidelines provide clear direction.

Intermediate scenarios introduce multi-system involvement and require prioritization skills. Here, you'll encounter patients with competing needs, where multiple problems demand your attention simultaneously. These scenarios challenge you to move beyond protocol-driven thinking toward more nuanced clinical reasoning.

Advanced scenarios present complex multi-system cases requiring leadership skills and ethical considerations. These situations mirror the most challenging aspects of nursing practice, where guidelines may conflict, resources are limited, and you must make difficult decisions under pressure.

Each scenario includes detailed patient presentations, progressive clinical data that unfolds as real situations do, decision points aligned with the CJMM framework, and NGN-style questions that mirror the current examination format. The rationales don't just explain correct answers—they walk you through the thinking process that leads to sound clinical judgment.

Using Scenarios Effectively

Effective use of these scenarios requires active engagement, not passive reading. Before jumping to the questions, spend time with each patient presentation. What stands out to you? What concerns you most? What additional information do you need? This preliminary analysis mirrors the clinical reality where you must form impressions and generate hypotheses before having complete information.

Work through scenarios in order within each level, but feel free to revisit earlier scenarios as you progress. You'll often find that your analysis becomes more sophisticated as your clinical judgment develops. A scenario that seemed straightforward initially may reveal new layers of complexity as your expertise grows.

Consider keeping a clinical judgment journal as you work through scenarios. Document your initial impressions, the reasoning behind your decisions, and your reflections after reviewing the rationales. This practice strengthens metacognitive skills—your ability to think about your thinking—which research shows correlates strongly with clinical judgment development (4).

Key Terms and Concepts

Understanding the language of clinical judgment helps clarify what we're actually trying to develop. **Clinical judgment** refers to the iterative process of noticing, interpreting, and responding to patient situations. It's dynamic, contextual, and improves with experience and reflection.

Critical thinking, while related, represents a broader cognitive skill set that includes analysis, evaluation, and logical reasoning. Clinical judgment applies critical thinking specifically to patient care situations, incorporating nursing knowledge, patient preferences, and contextual factors.

Clinical reasoning describes the cognitive processes underlying clinical judgment—how you move from noticing patient cues to taking appropriate action. It includes both analytical reasoning (systematic, rule-based thinking) and intuitive reasoning (pattern recognition based on experience).

The NGN introduces several new item types designed to assess these cognitive processes:

Bowtie questions present a central patient problem with branching decision points for assessment and intervention. These items test your ability to connect patient presentations with appropriate responses.

Trend questions require you to analyze patterns in patient data over time, reflecting the reality that patient conditions change and your interventions must adapt accordingly.

Matrix questions present multiple response options in grid format, allowing assessment of complex clinical scenarios with multiple correct responses.

Drag-and-drop items test your ability to sequence actions appropriately or match interventions with patient needs, reflecting the prioritization skills essential to clinical practice.

Complexity Indicators

Understanding complexity indicators helps you recognize when situations require heightened attention and more sophisticated clinical reasoning. Simple scenarios typically involve single problems with clear solutions, stable patient conditions, and well-established protocols. Complex scenarios involve multiple interacting problems, rapidly changing conditions, conflicting priorities, and situations where standard protocols may not apply directly.

For example, administrating scheduled medications to a stable patient represents a relatively simple scenario, but administrating those same medications when the patient develops new symptoms, shows signs of drug interactions, or expresses concerns about side effects introduces multiple layers of complexity.

Recognition of complexity indicators helps you adjust your clinical reasoning approach. Simple situations may require primarily analytical thinking, following established protocols and guidelines. Complex situations demand more intuitive reasoning, pattern recognition, and the ability to adapt when standard approaches don't fit perfectly.

Learning Through Cases

Let me walk you through how clinical judgment develops using three brief examples that illustrate different complexity levels:

Case Example 1: Basic Level Mrs. Johnson, 72, presents with blood pressure readings of 168/92 on three separate occasions. She has no other symptoms and her physical assessment is otherwise normal. In this straightforward scenario, you recognize elevated blood pressure as your primary cue, analyze it in the context of her age and absence of other symptoms, and prioritize hypertension management as your primary hypothesis. Your solution involves lifestyle counseling and medication management, actions include patient education and medication administration, and you evaluate outcomes by monitoring subsequent blood pressure readings.

Case Example 2: Intermediate Level Mr. Rodriguez, 65, presents with chest discomfort, diaphoresis, and nausea. His blood pressure is 180/98, heart rate 102, and he appears anxious. He has a history of diabetes and hyperlipidemia. Here, you recognize multiple cues that could indicate several conditions. Your analysis must consider the constellation of symptoms, not just individual findings. You prioritize acute coronary syndrome as your primary hypothesis while remaining alert to other possibilities. Your solutions include immediate interventions like obtaining an EKG, administrating aspirin, and preparing for potential emergency procedures.

Case Example 3: Advanced Level Mrs. Chen, 78, presents with altered mental status, fever, elevated white blood cell count, and hypotension. She has multiple chronic conditions including heart failure, diabetes, and chronic kidney disease. She takes twelve different medications. This complex scenario requires you to recognize subtle cues of sepsis while considering how her chronic conditions complicate both her presentation and your interventions. Your analysis must account for multiple interacting systems, your prioritization must balance competing needs, and your solutions must consider not just immediate stabilization but also how interventions might affect her other conditions.

Notice how complexity increases not just in terms of the number of problems, but in the degree of interaction between problems, the ambiguity of presentations, and the need to balance competing priorities.

Moving Forward

Clinical judgment development is neither linear nor predictable. Some days you'll feel confident in your decision-making abilities, while others will challenge every assumption you've made about patient care. This variability is normal and actually indicates healthy professional growth. Experts don't have all the answers—they've simply developed better strategies for managing uncertainty and learning from each clinical encounter.

The scenarios in this book provide a safe space to practice these cognitive skills before you encounter similar situations in clinical practice. They allow you to make mistakes, explore different approaches, and develop the pattern recognition that characterizes expert clinical judgment. Use them not just to prepare for examinations, but to build the thinking skills that will serve you throughout your nursing career.

Key Learning Points

- Clinical judgment represents the application of critical thinking to patient care situations

- The NGN reflects evidence-based recognition that traditional testing methods didn't adequately assess clinical reasoning skills

- Progressive complexity in scenarios mirrors natural learning progression from novice to expert

- Effective scenario use requires active engagement, reflection, and metacognitive awareness

- Complexity indicators help you recognize when situations require more sophisticated clinical reasoning approaches

- Clinical judgment development is iterative, contextual, and improves with practice and experience

Chapter 2: NCSBN Clinical Judgment Measurement Model (CJMM)

The Clinical Judgment Measurement Model didn't emerge from theoretical speculation—it grew from extensive research into how nurses actually think and make decisions in clinical practice. This framework provides a roadmap for understanding the cognitive processes that separate novice thinking from expert clinical judgment.

The Six Cognitive Functions

The CJMM identifies six distinct but interconnected cognitive functions that nurses use when making clinical decisions. These functions don't always occur in linear sequence—expert nurses often cycle through them rapidly and sometimes simultaneously. However, understanding each function helps you develop more systematic approaches to clinical reasoning.

Recognize Cues

Recognizing cues involves identifying relevant clinical information from the vast amount of data available in any patient encounter. This sounds simpler than it actually is. Novice nurses often struggle with what researchers call "cue saturation"—becoming overwhelmed by the sheer volume of available information and unable to distinguish between relevant and irrelevant data (5).

Effective cue recognition requires both knowledge and experience. You need to know what normal looks like before you can recognize abnormal findings. You also need experience with similar patients to develop pattern recognition skills that allow you to quickly identify significant changes or concerning findings.

Consider this scenario: You walk into a patient's room and immediately notice multiple pieces of information—the cardiac monitor shows sinus rhythm at 88 beats per minute, the patient is sitting up in bed watching television, the IV is infusing without signs of infiltration, the urinary catheter bag contains 200 mL of clear yellow urine, and the patient greets you with "Good morning, nurse."

A novice might try to process all this information equally, but an experienced nurse immediately recognizes that the normal greeting, alert demeanor, and stable vital signs suggest the patient is currently stable. This allows the nurse to focus attention on other priorities rather than conducting an unnecessarily detailed assessment of this stable patient.

Case Example: Cue Recognition in Action Maria Santos, a 68-year-old woman admitted for pneumonia, rings her call light at 0300. You enter her room and observe: she's sitting on the edge of the bed, breathing appears slightly labored with respirations at 24 per minute, oxygen saturation reads 89% on 2L nasal cannula (down from 94% at midnight), she's alert and oriented, skin feels warm and dry, and she states "I just can't seem to catch my breath."

The relevant cues here include the decreased oxygen saturation, increased respiratory rate, patient's subjective complaint of dyspnea, and the change from her baseline status. Less relevant cues include her alertness and orientation (important for overall assessment but not immediately related to her respiratory distress) and the warm, dry skin (which might be relevant if you suspected fever, but isn't directly related to her primary complaint).

Expert nurses develop what researchers call "clinical grasp"—the ability to quickly identify the most significant cues in complex situations (6). This skill develops through experience with similar patients and reflection on clinical encounters.

Analyze Cues

Analyzing cues involves making sense of the information you've recognized as relevant. This cognitive function requires you to connect patient data with your nursing knowledge to understand what might be happening with your patient.

Analysis occurs at different levels. Surface-level analysis might recognize that increased respiratory rate and decreased oxygen saturation suggest respiratory distress. Deeper analysis considers why this might be happening—is this progression of the patient's pneumonia, development of a complication like pneumothorax, or perhaps a different problem entirely?

Effective cue analysis requires both deductive reasoning (applying general principles to specific situations) and inductive reasoning (drawing general conclusions from specific observations). You use deductive reasoning when you apply your knowledge of pneumonia pathophysiology to understand why your patient might be experiencing respiratory distress. You use inductive reasoning when you notice patterns in your patient's presentation that suggest specific complications or conditions.

Case Example: Cue Analysis Development Returning to Maria Santos, analysis of her cues might proceed as follows: The decreased oxygen saturation combined with increased respiratory rate and subjective dyspnea suggests worsening respiratory status. Given her diagnosis of pneumonia, this could represent disease progression, development of pleural effusion, or another pulmonary complication. The timing (middle of the night) and acute onset suggest this represents a change from her baseline rather than expected disease progression.

Your analysis must also consider alternative explanations. Could she be experiencing cardiac complications? Pulmonary embolism? Anxiety? Effective analysis considers multiple possibilities while focusing on the most likely and most dangerous potential causes.

Prioritize Hypotheses

Prioritizing hypotheses involves ranking potential explanations for your patient's condition based on likelihood, urgency, and potential for harm. This cognitive function separates novice thinking from expert clinical judgment more than any other.

Novices often struggle with hypothesis prioritization because they treat all possible explanations as equally likely. Experts use probabilistic thinking, considering not just what could be causing a patient's symptoms, but what is most likely given the specific patient, context, and presenting pattern.

Prioritization also involves considering the consequences of being wrong. A hypothesis that, if correct, could result in serious harm requires immediate attention even if it's not the most likely explanation. This concept, borrowed from emergency medicine, is called "worst-case scenario thinking" and represents a crucial component of safe clinical practice (7).

Case Example: Hypothesis Prioritization in Practice For Maria Santos, your hypothesis prioritization might include:

1. **Highest priority**: Progression of pneumonia with increasing respiratory failure—most likely given her diagnosis and presentation, and requires immediate intervention

2. **High priority**: Pleural effusion—less likely but serious complication that would require urgent intervention

3. **Moderate priority**: Pulmonary embolism—less likely given her presentation pattern but potentially life-threatening

4. **Lower priority**: Anxiety-related dyspnea—possible but less likely given objective findings

This prioritization guides your immediate actions. You'll focus first on interventions for respiratory distress and pneumonia progression while remaining alert for signs that might suggest other conditions.

Generate Solutions

Generating solutions involves developing plans for addressing your patient's identified problems. This function requires you to connect your clinical knowledge with evidence-based interventions while considering your patient's specific circumstances, preferences, and resources.

Solution generation operates at multiple levels. Immediate solutions address urgent patient needs, intermediate solutions focus on ongoing management, and long-term solutions consider discharge

11

planning and patient education needs. Expert nurses seamlessly integrate all three levels when developing care plans.

Effective solution generation also requires considering multiple intervention options and selecting approaches most likely to be effective for your specific patient. Cookie-cutter approaches rarely work in complex clinical situations—interventions must be tailored to individual patient needs and circumstances.

Case Example: Solution Generation Process For Maria Santos, your solution generation might include:

Immediate interventions: Increase oxygen to maintain saturation above 92%, position patient for optimal breathing, assess lung sounds and respiratory effort more thoroughly, notify physician of status change, consider need for arterial blood gas analysis

Intermediate interventions: Monitor respiratory status closely, ensure adequate hydration, administer prescribed medications as appropriate, prepare for possible escalation of care

Long-term considerations: Patient education about pneumonia recovery, respiratory therapy consultation, discharge planning modifications based on current status

Take Action

Taking action involves implementing your chosen interventions while monitoring patient responses and remaining prepared to modify your approach based on outcomes. This function requires not just technical skills, but the ability to multitask, prioritize competing demands, and adapt quickly when situations change.

Effective action-taking also involves communication with other team members, documentation of interventions and patient responses, and coordination of care across multiple disciplines. Nurses rarely work in isolation—clinical judgment must account for team dynamics and resource availability.

Case Example: Action Implementation Your actions for Maria Santos might unfold as follows: You immediately increase her oxygen to 4L nasal cannula and help her into a more upright position. While she's adjusting to these changes, you listen to her lung sounds (noting increased crackles in the right lower lobe) and take a complete set of vital signs. You then call her physician to report the change in status, document your findings and interventions, and continue monitoring her response to your interventions.

Throughout this process, you're observing her responses and prepared to modify your approach if her condition doesn't improve or if it worsens further.

Evaluate Outcomes

Evaluating outcomes involves assessing the effectiveness of your interventions and determining next steps based on patient responses. This function closes the clinical judgment loop and often triggers repetition of the entire process as patient conditions change.

Outcome evaluation requires you to establish clear indicators for intervention success, monitor these indicators systematically, and recognize when alternative approaches are needed. Expert nurses develop sophisticated mental models for expected patient responses and quickly recognize when reality doesn't match expectations.

Case Example: Outcome Evaluation Twenty minutes after your interventions, Maria's oxygen saturation has improved to 92%, her respiratory rate has decreased to 20, and she reports feeling "a little better." These positive responses suggest your interventions were appropriate and effective. However, you continue monitoring because her response, while improved, isn't optimal. You might consider whether additional interventions are needed or whether you should prepare for possible escalation of care.

CJMM Layers and Context

The CJMM conceptualizes clinical judgment as occurring within multiple contextual layers that influence every decision you make.

Understanding these layers helps you recognize why identical patient presentations might require different approaches in different situations.

Layer 0: Clinical Decision Making represents the broadest context within which all clinical judgment occurs. This includes healthcare system factors, regulatory requirements, professional standards, and organizational policies that shape every patient encounter.

Layer 1: Clinical Judgment Process encompasses the specific context of individual patient encounters, including time pressures, resource availability, team dynamics, and environmental factors that influence your decision-making process.

Layer 2: Hypothesis Formation and Refinement involves the iterative process of developing and testing explanations for patient presentations. This layer reflects the reality that clinical judgment is rarely a one-time decision but rather an ongoing process of hypothesis testing and refinement.

Layer 3: Six Cognitive Functions represents the core framework we've discussed—the specific mental processes involved in clinical reasoning.

Layer 4: Environmental and Individual Factors includes both patient-specific factors (age, comorbidities, cultural background, preferences) and nurse-specific factors (experience level, knowledge base, fatigue, stress) that influence every clinical decision.

Applying CJMM to Clinical Practice

The CJMM provides a framework for understanding clinical judgment, but its real value lies in practical application. You can use this model to structure your thinking during patient encounters, reflect on your decision-making after clinical experiences, and identify areas for improvement in your clinical reasoning skills.

During patient encounters, consciously working through the six cognitive functions helps ensure you don't skip important steps in your reasoning process. This is particularly helpful in complex or stressful situations where it's easy to jump to conclusions or focus too narrowly on obvious problems while missing subtle but important changes.

Case Example: CJMM Application in Complex Situations Consider James Miller, a 45-year-old admitted for alcohol withdrawal who begins showing signs of confusion and agitation on his second hospital day. Using the CJMM framework:

Recognize Cues: Increased confusion (change from baseline), agitation, diaphoresis, tremors, elevated heart rate and blood pressure, patient stating he "sees things crawling on the walls"

Analyze Cues: These findings are consistent with progression of alcohol withdrawal, possibly developing into delirium tremens, a life-threatening complication. The hallucinations and autonomic instability are particularly concerning.

Prioritize Hypotheses: Delirium tremens is your highest priority hypothesis given the potential for seizures, cardiovascular collapse, and death. Alternative hypotheses include other causes of delirium (infection, metabolic disturbances) but are less likely given the context.

Generate Solutions: Immediate interventions include ensuring patient safety, administering prescribed benzodiazepines per protocol, continuous monitoring, physician notification, and preparation for possible intensive care transfer.

Take Action: Implement safety measures, administer medications, notify physician, begin close monitoring, and prepare for potential complications.

Evaluate Outcomes: Monitor patient response to interventions, watch for signs of improvement or deterioration, and be prepared to escalate care if his condition doesn't improve.

Common Pitfalls and Misconceptions

Several common errors can derail clinical judgment development. **Premature closure** occurs when you settle on a diagnosis or explanation too quickly, before gathering sufficient information or considering alternative possibilities. This error is particularly common when patients present with classic symptoms of common conditions—you assume the obvious explanation is correct without considering other possibilities.

Anchoring bias involves becoming too attached to your initial impression and failing to modify your thinking when new information becomes available. If you initially think a patient's symptoms represent a specific condition, you might interpret all subsequent information through that lens rather than remaining open to alternative explanations.

Confirmation bias leads you to seek information that supports your initial hypothesis while ignoring or downplaying information that contradicts it. This bias can prevent you from recognizing when your initial assessment was incorrect or incomplete.

Overconfidence in your clinical judgment can lead to inadequate information gathering, failure to seek consultation when appropriate, or reluctance to modify your approach when interventions aren't working as expected.

Self-Evaluation Using CJMM Framework

Regular self-evaluation using the CJMM framework strengthens your clinical reasoning skills and helps identify areas for improvement. After each significant patient encounter, consider walking through each cognitive function:

- What cues did I recognize, and what did I miss?

- How effectively did I analyze the information I gathered?

- Were my hypothesis priorities appropriate given the patient's presentation and context?

- Did my solutions address the most important patient needs?

- Were my actions timely, appropriate, and well-coordinated?

- How effectively did I evaluate outcomes and modify my approach based on patient responses?

This type of systematic reflection, while time-consuming initially, becomes second nature with practice and significantly accelerates clinical judgment development.

Building Expertise Through Deliberate Practice

Clinical judgment expertise develops through what researchers call "deliberate practice"—focused, effortful practice aimed at improving specific aspects of performance (8). Simply accumulating clinical experience isn't enough—you must actively work on improving your clinical reasoning skills.

The scenarios in this book provide opportunities for deliberate practice in clinical judgment. Use them not just to test your knowledge, but to practice systematic clinical reasoning. Work through each cognitive function deliberately, reflect on your thinking process, and identify patterns in your reasoning strengths and weaknesses.

Closing Thoughts

The CJMM provides more than just a theoretical framework—it offers a practical roadmap for developing the clinical reasoning skills that characterize expert nursing practice. These cognitive functions become automatic with experience, but initially require conscious effort and systematic practice.

The six cognitive functions work together in complex, often simultaneous ways that mirror the reality of clinical practice. Mastering them individually is important, but learning to integrate them seamlessly represents the hallmark of expert clinical judgment. The scenarios that follow provide structured opportunities to practice this integration in progressively complex situations that mirror real clinical practice.

Key Learning Points

- The CJMM identifies six cognitive functions that nurses use in clinical decision-making: recognize cues, analyze cues, prioritize hypotheses, generate solutions, take action, and evaluate outcomes

- These functions operate within multiple contextual layers that influence every clinical decision

- Effective cue recognition requires distinguishing relevant from irrelevant information in complex clinical situations

- Hypothesis prioritization involves probabilistic thinking and consideration of potential consequences

- Common cognitive biases can derail clinical judgment development if not recognized and addressed

- Deliberate practice using systematic reflection accelerates clinical reasoning skill development

- The CJMM provides a practical framework for both clinical decision-making and self-evaluation of reasoning skills

Chapter 3: Next Generation NCLEX Question Formats

The Next Generation NCLEX introduces question formats specifically designed to assess clinical judgment rather than simple recall or basic application of nursing knowledge. These new formats mirror the complexity of real clinical decision-making and require different test-taking strategies than traditional multiple-choice questions.

Understanding these formats isn't just about passing an examination—it's about developing the kind of thinking that will serve you well in clinical practice. The NGN question types reflect how nurses actually process information and make decisions in patient care situations.

Stand-Alone Items

Stand-alone NGN items present complete clinical scenarios with enhanced question formats that allow more sophisticated assessment of clinical reasoning. Unlike traditional questions that typically have one correct answer, these items often have multiple acceptable responses or require you to demonstrate understanding of relationships between patient data and nursing interventions.

Bowtie Questions

Bowtie questions present the most innovative format in the NGN examination. They're called "bowtie" because of their visual structure—a central patient problem with branching assessment parameters on one side and potential interventions on the other, connected by the nurse's clinical judgment.

These questions assess your ability to connect patient presentations with appropriate nursing responses. The left side typically presents potential assessment findings or risk factors, while the right side shows possible interventions. Your job is to identify which assessments are most relevant to the patient's condition and which interventions are most appropriate for addressing identified problems.

Bowtie questions reflect clinical reality more accurately than traditional formats. In practice, you don't just select one intervention for a patient problem—you implement multiple, coordinated interventions while monitoring various assessment parameters. The bowtie format allows assessment of this more complex clinical reasoning process.

Case Example: Bowtie Question Structure Consider a patient with heart failure exacerbation. A bowtie question might present various assessment parameters (daily weight, lung sounds, peripheral edema, blood pressure, urine output, oxygen saturation, heart rate) on the left side and potential interventions (oxygen therapy, diuretic administration, daily weights, fluid restriction, activity limitation, patient education) on the right side.

Your task involves identifying which assessments are most crucial for monitoring this patient's condition and which interventions are most appropriate for managing heart failure exacerbation. This requires understanding both the pathophysiology of heart failure and the nursing interventions most likely to improve patient outcomes.

The complexity of bowtie questions varies based on the clinical scenario. Simple bowtie items might focus on straightforward patient problems with clear assessment and intervention priorities. Complex bowtie items present patients with multiple interacting problems where assessment and intervention priorities are less obvious and require more sophisticated clinical reasoning.

Trend Questions

Trend questions require you to analyze patterns in patient data over time, reflecting the reality that patient conditions change and nursing care must adapt accordingly. These questions present data points across multiple time periods and ask you to identify significant patterns or predict likely outcomes based on observed trends.

Trend analysis represents a crucial component of clinical judgment that traditional question formats couldn't assess effectively. In practice, you constantly monitor how patients respond to interventions, recognize when conditions are improving or deteriorating, and modify care plans based on observed changes.

Case Example: Trend Question Application A trend question might present vital signs data for a post-operative patient across several time points: immediately post-op, 2 hours post-op, 4 hours post-op, and 6 hours post-op. The data might show gradually increasing heart rate, slowly decreasing blood pressure, stable temperature, and decreasing urine output.

Your analysis of this trend should recognize signs of possible hypovolemia or bleeding, understand that the pattern suggests clinical deterioration rather than normal post-operative recovery, and identify appropriate nursing interventions for addressing the suspected problem.

Trend questions can present various types of data—vital signs, laboratory values, pain scores, mobility assessments, or patient self-report measures. The key skill being assessed is your ability to recognize significant patterns and understand their clinical implications.

Practice Examples with Rationales

Let me walk you through detailed examples of each major NGN format to demonstrate how these questions assess clinical judgment:

Bowtie Example: COPD Exacerbation Patient scenario: Robert Chen, 68 years old, presents to the emergency department with increased shortness of breath, productive cough with yellow-green sputum, and fatigue. He has a 40-year history of cigarette smoking and known COPD. His current vital signs show: Temperature 100.8°F, Heart rate 108, Respirations 28, Blood pressure 158/92, Oxygen saturation 88% on room air.

Assessment parameters to consider: Sputum characteristics, breath sounds, use of accessory muscles, level of consciousness, skin color, capillary refill, arterial blood gas values, chest X-ray findings.

Potential interventions: Oxygen therapy, bronchodilator administration, corticosteroid therapy, antibiotics, chest physiotherapy, patient positioning, activity modification, patient education.

Your clinical judgment should identify sputum characteristics, breath sounds, and arterial blood gas values as priority assessments because they directly relate to respiratory function and infection status. Priority interventions should include oxygen therapy to address hypoxemia, bronchodilators for bronchospasm, and antibiotics for the suspected respiratory infection indicated by fever and purulent sputum.

Trend Example: Diabetic Ketoacidosis Management A 24-year-old patient with Type 1 diabetes is being treated for diabetic ketoacidosis. Review the following data trends over 6 hours of treatment:

Time 0000: Blood glucose 485 mg/dL, pH 7.18, Bicarbonate 12 mEq/L, Ketones 4+ Time 0200: Blood glucose 380 mg/dL, pH 7.22, Bicarbonate 14 mEq/L, Ketones 3+ Time 0400: Blood glucose 290 mg/dL, pH 7.28, Bicarbonate 16 mEq/L, Ketones 2+ Time 0600: Blood glucose 210 mg/dL, pH 7.35, Bicarbonate 18 mEq/L, Ketones 1+

This trend shows appropriate response to DKA treatment— decreasing glucose levels, improving pH and bicarbonate levels, and clearing ketones. The pattern suggests the treatment plan is effective and the patient is recovering from ketoacidosis. However, you should recognize that continued monitoring is essential because rapid glucose correction can lead to complications like cerebral edema.

Case Study Items

Case study items present more complex clinical scenarios that unfold over time, similar to how patient conditions actually develop in clinical practice. These items typically include multiple related questions that assess different aspects of clinical judgment within the same patient scenario.

Matrix/Grid Questions

Matrix questions present information in a grid format where you must select multiple appropriate responses from various categories. These questions recognize that patient care rarely involves single interventions—instead, you typically implement multiple coordinated actions to address patient needs comprehensively.

Matrix questions can assess various aspects of clinical judgment. Some focus on prioritization, asking you to rank interventions in order of importance. Others assess comprehensiveness, requiring you to identify all appropriate interventions for a given patient situation. Still others test discrimination, asking you to differentiate between appropriate and inappropriate actions for specific patients.

Case Example: Matrix Question Format A matrix question for a patient with pneumonia might present a grid with various potential nursing actions and ask you to categorize them as "immediate priority," "important but not immediate," or "not indicated." The actions might include: oxygen therapy, antibiotic administration, pain management, patient education, mobility assessment, nutritional evaluation, discharge planning, and spiritual care referral.

Your clinical judgment should identify oxygen therapy and antibiotic administration as immediate priorities because they directly address the patient's respiratory compromise and infection. Patient education and mobility assessment might be important but not immediate priorities, while discharge planning might be premature for an acutely ill patient.

Drag-and-Drop Questions

Drag-and-drop questions require you to sequence actions appropriately or match interventions with patient needs. These formats assess your understanding of proper procedure sequences, prioritization of multiple interventions, or connections between patient problems and appropriate nursing responses.

Cloze variations present scenarios with missing information that you must fill in by dragging appropriate options into blank spaces. These questions often assess medication knowledge, patient education content, or care planning decisions.

Rationale drag-and-drop questions require you to match interventions with their underlying rationales, testing your understanding of the reasoning behind nursing actions rather than just the actions themselves.

Case Example: Drag-and-Drop Sequencing A drag-and-drop question might ask you to sequence the steps for managing a patient experiencing chest pain:

Available actions: Obtain 12-lead EKG, administer oxygen, assess vital signs, notify physician, administer prescribed nitroglycerin, position patient comfortably, obtain focused history, initiate IV access.

The appropriate sequence prioritizes immediate life-threatening concerns first: position patient comfortably and administer oxygen for symptom relief, assess vital signs for baseline data, obtain 12-lead EKG for diagnostic information, notify physician with findings, then implement ordered interventions like nitroglycerin and IV access.

Highlighting Items

Highlighting questions ask you to identify relevant information within text passages or data tables. These questions assess your ability to recognize important clinical cues within complex presentations, mirroring the real-world skill of identifying significant information among large amounts of patient data.

Text highlighting questions present patient scenarios or documentation and ask you to highlight information that supports specific conclusions or indicates particular patient problems. These questions test cue recognition skills within realistic clinical documentation.

Table highlighting questions present data in tabular format and ask you to identify relevant values or concerning trends. These might include laboratory results, vital signs data, or medication administration records.

Case Example: Text Highlighting A highlighting question might present this documentation: "Patient states 'I've been having this nagging chest discomfort for the past three days, especially when I walk upstairs to my bedroom. It feels like pressure, not really pain, and it goes away when I sit down and rest for a few minutes. I've also been more tired than usual and had to stop twice going up the stairs today, which never happened before.'"

You might be asked to highlight information that suggests possible cardiac problems. Relevant highlighting would include: "chest discomfort," "especially when I walk upstairs," "pressure," "goes away when I sit down and rest," and "more tired than usual." This information suggests exertional angina and decreased exercise tolerance, both concerning for cardiac problems.

Unfolding Case Study Structure

Unfolding case studies present the most complex NGN format, reflecting how patient situations actually develop over time in clinical practice. These cases begin with initial patient presentations and then provide additional information at timed intervals, requiring you to modify your clinical reasoning as new data becomes available.

Unfolding cases assess your ability to adapt your thinking when patient conditions change, recognize when initial interventions aren't effective, and modify care plans based on new information. This flexibility in clinical reasoning represents a hallmark of expert nursing judgment.

Case Example: Unfolding Case Development An unfolding case might begin with a 45-year-old woman presenting to the emergency department with abdominal pain. Initial questions assess your ability to recognize relevant cues, prioritize assessments, and plan initial interventions.

The case then unfolds with additional information: laboratory results show elevated white blood cell count and positive pregnancy test, ultrasound reveals no intrauterine pregnancy, and the patient's pain has worsened and localized to the right lower quadrant.

Later questions assess your ability to modify your initial hypotheses (from general abdominal pain to possible ectopic pregnancy), reprioritize interventions (from routine pain management to emergency surgical preparation), and adapt your care plan based on changing patient status.

Scoring Methods and Test Strategy

Understanding NGN scoring helps you approach these questions strategically. Unlike traditional NCLEX questions that use simple right/wrong scoring, NGN items use more sophisticated scoring methods that provide partial credit for partially correct responses.

0/1 scoring applies to questions with single correct answers, similar to traditional NCLEX questions. You receive full credit for correct responses and no credit for incorrect responses.

+/- scoring (partial credit) applies to questions with multiple correct responses or multiple components. You receive positive points for correct selections and negative points for incorrect selections, with your total score reflecting the overall accuracy of your response.

Rationale scoring evaluates not just your answer selections but also your reasoning for those selections. Some NGN items ask you to explain your thinking or match interventions with their rationales, providing more comprehensive assessment of your clinical judgment process.

Time Management Strategies

NGN questions typically require more time than traditional multiple-choice items because they assess more complex cognitive processes.

Effective time management involves balancing thoroughness with efficiency—you need enough time to analyze complex scenarios carefully without spending so much time on individual questions that you can't complete the examination.

Read scenarios completely before attempting to answer questions. NGN scenarios often contain crucial information throughout the entire presentation, and premature answering based on incomplete information frequently leads to incorrect responses.

Use the scratch paper strategically to organize your thinking. For complex scenarios, jotting down key patient problems, priority assessments, or intervention sequences can help you work through questions systematically.

Practice pattern recognition with various NGN formats so you quickly understand what each question type is assessing. Familiarity with question formats allows you to focus your cognitive energy on clinical reasoning rather than figuring out how to approach unfamiliar question structures.

Approaching Different Item Types

Each NGN format requires slightly different cognitive approaches:

For bowtie questions, systematically consider the relationships between patient problems, relevant assessments, and appropriate interventions. Don't just select assessments and interventions in isolation—think about how they connect to address the patient's specific problems.

For trend questions, look for patterns rather than focusing on individual data points. Consider what the overall pattern suggests about the patient's condition and response to treatment.

For matrix questions, think comprehensively about patient needs and systematically consider each potential intervention's appropriateness and priority level.

For drag-and-drop questions, consider logical sequences and relationships. Think about what must happen first, what can happen simultaneously, and what should happen in what order.

For highlighting questions, focus on information that directly relates to the specific clinical question being asked. Avoid highlighting interesting but irrelevant information.

Preparing for Success

Success with NGN formats requires practice with clinical reasoning rather than memorization of facts. These questions assess your ability to think through patient situations systematically, not your ability to recall specific information.

Practice with realistic scenarios that mirror the complexity and ambiguity of actual patient care situations. The scenarios in this book are designed to provide this type of practice opportunity.

Develop systematic approaches to clinical reasoning that you can apply consistently across different patient situations. The CJMM framework provides an excellent structure for this systematic thinking.

Reflect on your reasoning process after working through practice scenarios. Understanding why you made specific decisions helps you identify patterns in your thinking and areas for improvement.

Synthesis and Moving Forward

The NGN question formats represent more than just new ways to ask test questions—they reflect a fundamental shift toward assessing the kind of thinking that characterizes safe, effective nursing practice. These formats require you to demonstrate clinical judgment skills that mirror real-world patient care situations.

Mastering these formats involves developing the underlying clinical reasoning skills they're designed to assess. Focus your preparation efforts on strengthening your ability to recognize relevant clinical cues, analyze patient data systematically, prioritize competing patient needs, generate appropriate solutions, and evaluate intervention effectiveness.

The investment you make in developing these skills will serve you well beyond any examination. The cognitive processes assessed by NGN questions represent the foundation of expert nursing practice—skills you'll use in every patient encounter throughout your nursing career.

Key Learning Points

- NGN question formats assess clinical judgment skills rather than simple recall or basic application

- Bowtie questions evaluate connections between patient problems, assessments, and interventions

- Trend questions assess pattern recognition and understanding of changes over time

- Matrix questions test comprehensive thinking about multiple patient needs and interventions

- Drag-and-drop items evaluate sequencing, prioritization, and matching skills

- Highlighting questions assess cue recognition within complex clinical presentations

- Unfolding cases mirror real-world patient situations that change over time

- Scoring methods include both traditional right/wrong and partial credit approaches

- Success requires systematic clinical reasoning skills rather than memorization

- These formats prepare you for the complexity of real clinical decision-making

Chapter 4: Building Clinical Judgment Skills

Clinical judgment doesn't develop overnight, and it certainly doesn't emerge automatically from accumulating clinical experiences. Research shows that some nurses with years of experience still struggle with complex clinical reasoning, while others develop sophisticated judgment skills relatively early in their careers. The difference lies not in the quantity of experience, but in how deliberately nurses work to develop their clinical reasoning abilities.

Novice to Expert Development

Patricia Benner's groundbreaking research identified five distinct stages of nursing competence development, each characterized by different approaches to clinical reasoning and decision-making (9). Understanding these stages helps you recognize your current level of development and identify specific skills to focus on as you progress toward expertise.

The Five Stages of Competence

Novice stage characterizes most nursing students and new graduates. Novice nurses rely heavily on rules and guidelines because they lack the experiential knowledge needed for more flexible clinical reasoning. This isn't a weakness—it's an appropriate and necessary stage of development. Novices need clear protocols and structured approaches to ensure safe patient care while they build foundational knowledge and begin developing pattern recognition skills.

Novice thinking is characterized by what researchers call "analytical reasoning"—systematic, step-by-step processing that follows established rules and procedures. While this approach can appear slow and inflexible, it provides crucial safeguards against errors when clinical experience is limited.

Case Example: Novice Clinical Reasoning Sarah, a new graduate nurse, encounters a patient complaining of chest pain. Her approach follows established protocols systematically: she positions the patient, applies oxygen, obtains vital signs, performs a 12-lead EKG, notifies the physician, and prepares for possible interventions. She follows each step methodically, consulting her reference materials to ensure she hasn't missed anything important.

While experienced nurses might accomplish these same tasks more quickly and fluidly, Sarah's systematic approach ensures thorough assessment and appropriate initial interventions. Her detailed documentation reflects her methodical reasoning process and provides excellent communication with other team members.

Advanced beginner stage develops after several months of clinical experience, when nurses begin recognizing recurring patterns in patient presentations but still rely heavily on guidelines and experienced nurses for decision-making support. Advanced beginners start developing what Benner calls "situated knowledge"— understanding that emerges from experience with real patients in specific contexts.

Advanced beginners begin recognizing when standard protocols might not fit perfectly with specific patient situations, but they often struggle with how to modify their approaches appropriately. This stage is characterized by increasing confidence tempered by growing awareness of clinical complexity.

Competent stage typically emerges after two to three years of practice in similar clinical situations. Competent nurses develop the ability to prioritize patient needs effectively, manage multiple patients simultaneously, and modify their approaches based on patient responses. They begin using both analytical and intuitive reasoning, though they still rely more heavily on analytical approaches for complex situations.

Competent nurses develop what researchers call "clinical grasp"—the ability to quickly identify the most significant aspects of complex patient presentations. They also begin developing forward-thinking skills, anticipating potential complications and preparing preventive interventions.

Case Example: Competent Clinical Reasoning Mark, a nurse with three years of experience, walks into a patient's room and immediately notices subtle changes in the patient's appearance and behavior that suggest early deterioration. His assessment focuses quickly on the most relevant parameters, and he implements interventions while simultaneously planning for potential complications. His documentation captures not just what he observed and did, but his reasoning for his actions and his plans for ongoing monitoring.

Proficient stage nurses have developed sophisticated pattern recognition skills that allow them to grasp complex patient situations holistically rather than analytically. They recognize when patient presentations don't fit typical patterns and modify their approaches accordingly. Proficient nurses use predominantly intuitive reasoning, shifting to analytical reasoning primarily when they encounter unfamiliar situations.

Proficient nurses also develop advanced communication skills, serving as resources for less experienced nurses and effectively collaborating with physicians and other healthcare team members. They often take on leadership roles and contribute to quality improvement initiatives.

Expert stage nurses demonstrate the most sophisticated clinical judgment skills, characterized by intuitive grasp of complex situations and the ability to focus immediately on the most relevant aspects of patient problems. Expert nurses have developed extensive repertoires of experiential knowledge that allow them to recognize subtle patterns and respond appropriately to unusual situations.

Expert nurses also demonstrate advanced ethical reasoning skills, effectively balancing competing patient needs, family concerns, and system constraints. They often serve as mentors and clinical leaders, contributing to the development of less experienced nurses.

Characteristics at Each Level

Understanding the specific characteristics of each developmental stage helps you assess your current level and identify areas for focused improvement. These characteristics aren't fixed—nurses may demonstrate different levels of competence in different clinical situations, and development isn't always linear.

Novice characteristics include: Reliance on rules and protocols, difficulty prioritizing when guidelines conflict, tendency to focus on individual tasks rather than holistic patient care, and need for significant guidance and support from experienced nurses.

Advanced beginner characteristics include: Beginning pattern recognition, increased confidence with routine patient care, occasional recognition that protocols might not fit specific situations, and continued need for support with complex decision-making.

Competent characteristics include: Effective prioritization skills, ability to manage multiple patients simultaneously, development of forward-thinking and anticipatory skills, and increasing independence in clinical decision-making.

Proficient characteristics include: Sophisticated pattern recognition, holistic approach to patient care, ability to modify approaches based on patient responses, and effective collaboration with interdisciplinary teams.

Expert characteristics include: Intuitive grasp of complex situations, ability to focus immediately on relevant aspects of patient problems, advanced ethical reasoning skills, and effectiveness in mentoring and leadership roles.

Progression Indicators

Several indicators suggest progression from one stage to the next. **Increasing efficiency** in patient care tasks often indicates developing pattern recognition and clinical grasp. **Growing comfort with ambiguity** suggests developing tolerance for the uncertainty inherent in clinical practice. **Improved prioritization skills** indicate advancing ability to manage multiple competing demands effectively.

Enhanced communication skills often accompany clinical judgment development, as nurses become better able to articulate their reasoning and collaborate effectively with team members. **Increased anticipatory thinking** suggests developing ability to predict potential complications and prepare preventive interventions.

Growing confidence balanced with appropriate humility indicates healthy professional development. Expert nurses are confident in their abilities while remaining open to learning and recognizing the limits of their knowledge.

Self-Assessment Tools

Regular self-assessment using structured tools accelerates clinical judgment development by promoting metacognitive awareness— thinking about your thinking. Several validated instruments can help you assess your current level of clinical reasoning development.

The **Lasater Clinical Judgment Rubric (LCJR)** provides detailed criteria for assessing clinical judgment skills across four dimensions: noticing, interpreting, responding, and reflecting (10). You can use this rubric to evaluate your performance in clinical situations and identify specific areas for improvement.

Reflective journaling provides another powerful tool for self-assessment and clinical judgment development. Structured reflection using frameworks like Johns' Model of Structured Reflection or Gibbs' Reflective Cycle helps you analyze clinical experiences systematically and extract learning from each patient encounter (11).

Peer feedback and **preceptor evaluation** provide external perspectives on your clinical reasoning development. Regular discussions with experienced nurses about your decision-making process can reveal blind spots and suggest areas for focused improvement.

Clinical Judgment Models

While Benner's novice-to-expert model describes developmental stages, other models focus on the specific cognitive processes involved in clinical judgment. Understanding these models provides additional frameworks for developing clinical reasoning skills.

Tanner's Clinical Judgment Model

Christine Tanner's Clinical Judgment Model identifies four phases of clinical reasoning: noticing, interpreting, responding, and reflecting (12). This model emphasizes the influence of background knowledge, experience, and contextual factors on every aspect of clinical judgment.

Noticing involves recognizing changes in patient status, identifying relevant clinical cues, and distinguishing between normal and abnormal findings. Effective noticing requires both theoretical knowledge and experiential knowledge that develops through caring for similar patients.

Interpreting involves making sense of noticed cues by connecting them with theoretical knowledge and experiential understanding. This phase includes developing hypotheses about patient problems and considering alternative explanations for patient presentations.

Responding involves implementing appropriate interventions based on your interpretation of patient situations. Effective responding requires not just knowledge of potential interventions, but understanding of which interventions are most appropriate for specific patients in particular contexts.

Reflecting involves evaluating the outcomes of your interventions and learning from each clinical experience. Reflection includes both reflection-in-action (adjusting your approach while caring for patients) and reflection-on-action (analyzing experiences after they occur).

Case Example: Tanner's Model in Practice Jennifer, working with a post-operative patient, notices (first phase) that the patient seems more restless than earlier and his surgical dressing has a small amount of bright red drainage. She interprets (second phase) these cues as potentially indicating bleeding, though she also considers alternative explanations like pain or anxiety. She responds (third phase) by assessing vital signs, examining the surgical site more thoroughly, and notifying the surgeon of her concerns. Later, she reflects (fourth phase) on the experience, considering what cues were most significant and how she might recognize similar situations more quickly in the future.

Lasater Clinical Judgment Rubric

The Lasater Clinical Judgment Rubric operationalizes Tanner's model by providing specific behavioral indicators for each phase of clinical judgment. This rubric helps assess clinical judgment development and provides concrete goals for improvement.

Noticing indicators include focused observation, recognizing deviations from expected patterns, and information seeking. Developing nurses progress from requiring prompts to notice relevant changes to independently recognizing subtle cues that suggest important patient status changes.

Interpreting indicators include prioritizing data, making sense of data, and calm, confident manner. Growth in this area involves increasing sophistication in data analysis and growing comfort with clinical uncertainty.

Responding indicators include calm, confident manner, clear communication, well-planned intervention, and skillful performance. Development involves increasing efficiency and effectiveness in intervention implementation.

Reflecting indicators include evaluation and self-analysis, commitment to improvement. Advanced reflecting involves sophisticated analysis of clinical decisions and systematic approaches to learning from experience.

Integration with CJMM

The Clinical Judgment Measurement Model integrates well with both Benner's developmental model and Tanner's process model. The six cognitive functions of the CJMM (recognize cues, analyze cues, prioritize hypotheses, generate solutions, take action, evaluate outcomes) provide specific focus areas for skill development within the broader frameworks provided by these other models.

Novice nurses might focus primarily on developing cue recognition and basic analysis skills, while more advanced nurses work on sophisticated hypothesis prioritization and solution generation. Expert nurses excel at all six functions and integrate them seamlessly in complex clinical situations.

Practical Application Strategies

Understanding theoretical models is helpful, but practical application strategies make the real difference in clinical judgment development. These strategies help you translate theoretical understanding into improved clinical reasoning skills.

Deliberate practice involves focused, effortful practice aimed at improving specific aspects of performance. Unlike routine practice, deliberate practice targets your areas of weakness and pushes you beyond your current comfort zone. The scenarios in this book provide opportunities for deliberate practice in clinical reasoning.

Case-based learning using realistic patient scenarios helps you develop pattern recognition skills and practice clinical reasoning in low-risk environments. Work through scenarios systematically, using frameworks like the CJMM or Tanner's model to structure your thinking.

Simulation experiences provide opportunities to practice clinical reasoning in realistic but safe environments. Take full advantage of simulation learning by preparing thoroughly, participating actively, and reflecting systematically on your performance.

Concept mapping helps you visualize relationships between patient problems, underlying pathophysiology, and appropriate interventions. Creating concept maps for complex patients helps you develop holistic thinking skills and understand connections between seemingly separate problems.

Effective Learning Strategies

Clinical judgment development requires more than just accumulating clinical experience—it requires intentional learning strategies that promote deep understanding and skill development.

Active Learning Principles

Active learning involves engaging with material in ways that promote understanding and retention rather than passive absorption of information. **Elaborative rehearsal** involves connecting new information with existing knowledge, creating rich networks of understanding that support clinical reasoning.

Spaced practice involves spreading learning activities over time rather than concentrating them in single sessions. Research shows that spaced practice promotes longer retention and better transfer to new situations than massed practice.

Interleaved practice involves mixing different types of problems rather than practicing one type at a time. This approach better prepares you for the unpredictability of clinical practice, where patient problems don't present in neat categories.

Case Example: Active Learning Application Rather than studying cardiac conditions by reading about each one separately, you might work through mixed scenarios involving various cardiac patients, forcing yourself to differentiate between different conditions and appropriate interventions. This interleaved approach better prepares you for clinical situations where you must quickly distinguish between different cardiac problems.

Reflection and Debriefing Techniques

Structured reflection using established frameworks helps you extract maximum learning from clinical experiences. The "What? So What?

Now What?" framework provides a simple but effective structure for reflection.

"What?" involves describing what happened during a clinical experience, including your observations, actions, and patient responses. Focus on objective description rather than interpretation during this phase.

"So What?" involves analyzing the experience, considering what went well, what could have been improved, and what you learned. This phase includes connecting the experience with theoretical knowledge and identifying patterns in your clinical reasoning.

"Now What?" involves planning how you'll apply what you learned to future clinical situations. This forward-looking phase helps ensure that reflection leads to actual improvement in clinical practice.

Group debriefing after clinical experiences provides opportunities to learn from peers' experiences and gain different perspectives on clinical situations. Effective debriefing requires psychological safety— an environment where participants feel comfortable sharing uncertainties and mistakes without fear of judgment.

Peer Collaboration Methods

Peer learning partnerships provide mutual support for clinical judgment development. Working with peers at similar developmental levels allows you to share experiences, compare reasoning processes, and learn from each other's perspectives.

Think-aloud protocols involve verbalizing your reasoning process while working through clinical scenarios. This technique helps you become more aware of your thinking patterns and allows peers to provide feedback on your reasoning process.

Case presentations to peers provide opportunities to practice articulating your clinical reasoning and receive feedback on your decision-making process. Regular case presentations help you develop confidence in your clinical judgment and improve your ability to communicate your reasoning to others.

Transfer to Clinical Practice

The ultimate goal of clinical judgment development is improved patient care in real clinical situations. **Transfer** involves applying knowledge and skills learned in one context to different but related contexts.

Near transfer involves applying clinical reasoning skills to similar patient situations. This type of transfer is relatively straightforward and occurs naturally as you gain experience with specific patient populations.

Far transfer involves applying clinical reasoning principles to very different patient situations or clinical contexts. This more challenging type of transfer requires deep understanding of underlying principles rather than surface-level pattern recognition.

Promoting transfer requires explicit connection-making between learning experiences and clinical practice. After working through scenarios or simulation experiences, consciously consider how the reasoning skills you practiced might apply to different patient situations you encounter in clinical practice.

Building Confidence and Competence

Clinical judgment development requires balancing confidence with appropriate humility. **Confidence** enables decisive action when patients need immediate intervention, while **humility** promotes continued learning and appropriate help-seeking when situations exceed your current capabilities.

Graduated exposure to increasingly complex clinical situations helps build confidence while maintaining safety. Start with straightforward patient assignments and gradually take on more complex cases as your skills develop.

Mentor relationships with experienced nurses provide guidance, support, and feedback during clinical judgment development. Effective mentors not only demonstrate expert clinical reasoning but also help you develop your own reasoning skills through questioning, coaching, and encouragement.

Constructive self-talk supports confidence development while maintaining realistic self-assessment. Replace self-critical internal dialogue with more balanced self-evaluation that acknowledges both strengths and areas for improvement.

Overcoming Common Obstacles

Several common obstacles can impede clinical judgment development. **Performance anxiety** can interfere with clinical reasoning by overwhelming working memory and narrowing attention. Developing anxiety management strategies helps maintain clear thinking during stressful clinical situations.

Imposter syndrome can undermine confidence and prevent you from taking appropriate clinical risks that promote growth. Remember that feeling uncertain or overwhelmed is normal during skill development—expertise takes time to develop.

Information overload can occur when you try to process too much information simultaneously. Developing systematic approaches to data gathering and analysis helps manage information more effectively.

Perfectionism can interfere with learning by making you overly cautious about making mistakes. Remember that errors are inevitable during learning and provide valuable opportunities for growth when analyzed constructively.

Sustaining Development

Clinical judgment development is a career-long process that requires sustained effort and commitment. **Lifelong learning** attitudes support continued growth throughout your nursing career.

Professional development activities like continuing education, certification programs, and advanced degree preparation provide structured opportunities for continued clinical reasoning skill development.

Quality improvement participation allows you to apply clinical reasoning skills to systems-level problems and contribute to improved patient outcomes beyond individual patient care.

Mentoring others provides opportunities to articulate your clinical reasoning and reflect on your own development while supporting the growth of less experienced nurses.

Closing Reflections

Clinical judgment development represents one of the most rewarding aspects of nursing practice. The ability to think through complex patient situations, make sound decisions under pressure, and adapt your approach based on patient responses provides both professional satisfaction and the foundation for excellent patient care.

The journey from novice to expert takes time, effort, and commitment, but the investment pays dividends throughout your nursing career. Each patient encounter provides opportunities to refine your clinical reasoning skills, and each reflection on your practice contributes to your growing expertise.

The frameworks and strategies discussed in this chapter provide roadmaps for development, but your actual growth will be unique to your experiences, learning style, and clinical context. Trust the process, be patient with yourself, and remain committed to continuous improvement. The nursing profession and the patients you serve will benefit from your dedication to developing expert clinical judgment skills.

Key Learning Points

- Clinical judgment develops through five distinct stages from novice to expert, each with characteristic reasoning approaches

- Tanner's Clinical Judgment Model identifies four phases: noticing, interpreting, responding, and reflecting

- The Lasater Clinical Judgment Rubric provides specific behavioral indicators for assessing clinical reasoning development

- Deliberate practice using structured scenarios accelerates skill development more than routine clinical experience alone

- Active learning strategies promote deeper understanding and better transfer to clinical practice

- Structured reflection using established frameworks maximizes learning from clinical experiences

- Peer collaboration provides mutual support and diverse perspectives on clinical reasoning

- Confidence development requires balancing decisiveness with appropriate humility and help-seeking

- Common obstacles include performance anxiety, imposter syndrome, information overload, and perfectionism

- Clinical judgment development is a career-long process requiring sustained commitment to learning and growth

Chapter 5: Progressive Medical-Surgical Scenarios

The scenarios that follow represent the heart of this book—carefully crafted patient situations designed to develop your clinical judgment skills systematically. These scenarios progress from straightforward single-system problems to complex multi-system cases that challenge even experienced nurses.

Understanding Scenario Progression

The progression from beginner to advanced scenarios mirrors the natural development of clinical expertise. Beginner scenarios focus on pattern recognition and protocol application—skills essential for safe practice but representing only the foundation of clinical judgment. Intermediate scenarios require prioritization and adaptation—hallmarks of competent nursing practice. Advanced scenarios demand sophisticated clinical reasoning, leadership skills, and the ability to manage competing priorities under pressure.

Each scenario includes multiple components designed to simulate real clinical encounters: comprehensive patient presentations, relevant background history, progressive clinical data that unfolds over time, decision points that mirror actual clinical reasoning, NGN-style questions that assess specific cognitive functions, and detailed rationales that explain not just correct answers but the thinking processes that lead to sound clinical judgment.

How to Use These Scenarios

Approach each scenario as you would a real patient encounter. Read the initial presentation carefully, forming preliminary impressions before looking at the questions. Consider what additional information you need, what concerns you most about this patient, and what your priorities might be for nursing care.

Work through the questions systematically, but don't just select answers—think about your reasoning process. What cues led you to specific conclusions? How did you prioritize competing patient needs? What alternatives did you consider? This metacognitive awareness—thinking about your thinking—accelerates clinical judgment development more than simply practicing questions.

After completing each scenario, spend time with the rationales. These explanations provide insights into expert clinical reasoning and help you understand not just what to do, but why and how expert nurses think through complex patient situations.

Chapter 6: Cardiovascular Scenarios

The beginner scenarios focus on developing fundamental clinical judgment skills using single-system problems with relatively clear presentations and established protocols. These scenarios help you practice recognizing relevant clinical cues, analyzing their significance, and implementing appropriate interventions while building confidence in your clinical reasoning abilities.

Scenario 1: Stable Hypertension Management

Patient Presentation: Margaret Torres, a 68-year-old retired teacher, presents to her primary care provider for routine follow-up. Three weeks ago, her blood pressure readings were 168/92, 172/88, and 165/90 on separate occasions. She was started on lisinopril 10 mg daily. Today, her vital signs show: Blood pressure 148/84, Heart rate 76, Respirations 18, Temperature 98.6°F, Oxygen saturation 98% on room air. She reports no symptoms and states she's been taking her medication as prescribed.

Mrs. Torres has a medical history of osteoarthritis and takes ibuprofen occasionally for joint pain. She denies tobacco use but admits to drinking two glasses of wine most evenings. Her BMI is 28. Family history includes hypertension in both parents and diabetes in her mother. She retired two years ago and describes her current stress level as "much better than when I was working."

Physical Assessment: Alert and oriented, pleasant demeanor, no acute distress. Cardiovascular examination reveals regular rate and rhythm, no murmurs or extra sounds, peripheral pulses intact bilaterally. Lung sounds clear throughout. Abdomen soft, non-tender. No peripheral edema noted.

Laboratory Results: Basic metabolic panel within normal limits, creatinine 0.9 mg/dL, potassium 4.2 mEq/L, sodium 140 mEq/L.

This scenario focuses on recognizing the cues of partially controlled hypertension, analyzing the factors that might influence blood pressure control, and planning appropriate interventions for ongoing management. The blood pressure reduction from previous readings suggests the medication is having some effect, but the values remain above target levels for her age group.

Key cues include the partially improved but still elevated blood pressure readings, the patient's medication adherence, lifestyle factors like wine consumption and occasional NSAID use, and the absence of symptoms. Analysis should consider the medication's partial effectiveness, potential lifestyle modifications, and the need for continued monitoring.

The prioritization here is straightforward—hypertension management takes precedence, but the patient's stability allows for a measured approach focusing on optimization of current therapy and lifestyle modifications rather than emergency interventions.

NGN-Style Questions:

Highlight the assessment findings that require nursing intervention: "Mrs. Torres reports taking her medication as prescribed, blood pressure readings show improvement from baseline but remain at 148/84, she occasionally uses ibuprofen for arthritis pain, and drinks two glasses of wine most evenings. She denies tobacco use and reports reduced stress since retirement."

The highlighted items should include the persistent elevation of blood pressure despite medication, the NSAID use which can interfere with ACE inhibitor effectiveness, and the alcohol consumption which can affect blood pressure control.

Rationale: The blood pressure reading of 148/84, while improved from initial readings in the 160s-170s systolic range, remains above recommended targets for adults (less than 130/80 for most adults, particularly those with cardiovascular risk factors). The occasional ibuprofen use represents a significant concern because NSAIDs can reduce the effectiveness of ACE inhibitors and contribute to elevated blood pressure. The two glasses of wine daily, while not excessive, can contribute to hypertension and should be addressed as part of comprehensive management.

Scenario 2: Routine Post-Cardiac Catheterization Care

Patient Presentation: David Kim, a 55-year-old accountant, returns to the medical unit following diagnostic cardiac catheterization via right femoral approach. The procedure was completed two hours ago without complications. Current vital signs: Blood pressure 132/78, Heart rate 68, Respirations 16, Temperature 98.4°F, Oxygen saturation 97% on room air.

Mr. Kim has a history of hyperlipidemia and family history of coronary artery disease. He presented to his cardiologist with atypical chest discomfort during exercise. The catheterization revealed minimal coronary disease not requiring intervention. He received conscious sedation during the procedure and is now alert and oriented.

Physical Assessment: Patient resting comfortably in bed with head of bed elevated 30 degrees. Right groin dressing dry and intact with no bleeding or hematoma noted. Distal pulses (dorsalis pedis and posterior tibial) palpable bilaterally. Skin warm and dry. No complaints of pain or discomfort. Foley catheter removed one hour ago; patient has not voided since the procedure.

Post-Procedure Orders: Bed rest with affected leg straight for 4 hours, vital signs every 15 minutes for first hour then every 30 minutes for 2 hours then hourly, assess groin site every 15 minutes for first hour then every hour, encourage oral fluids, ambulate after bed rest period if no complications.

This scenario focuses on recognizing normal post-catheterization recovery while remaining alert for potential complications. The patient's stability allows for routine post-procedure monitoring, but several assessment priorities require attention: access site integrity, distal circulation, and urinary function.

Key cues include the uncomplicated procedure, stable vital signs, intact access site without bleeding, present distal pulses, and the patient's comfort level. However, attention should be paid to the fact that he hasn't voided since catheter removal, which could indicate urinary retention or inadequate hydration.

NGN-Style Matrix Question: Categorize the following nursing actions as "High Priority," "Moderate Priority," or "Low Priority" for this patient:

Nursing Action	Priority Level
Assess groin site for bleeding	High Priority
Check distal pulses	High Priority
Encourage fluid intake	Moderate Priority
Assess for urinary retention	Moderate Priority
Pain assessment	Moderate Priority
Patient education about results	Low Priority
Ambulation preparation	Low Priority

Rationale: Access site assessment and distal pulse checks represent high priorities because bleeding or vascular compromise can occur suddenly and require immediate intervention. Fluid encouragement and urinary assessment are moderate priorities—important for preventing complications but not immediately life-threatening. Patient education and ambulation preparation are lower priorities until more critical assessments are completed and the patient has demonstrated stability through the required bed rest period.

Scenario 3: Stable Angina Education

Patient Presentation: Robert Chen, a 62-year-old engineer, was diagnosed with stable angina three months ago following cardiac catheterization that revealed 60% stenosis in his left anterior descending artery. He's being managed medically with atenolol 50 mg daily, atorvastatin 40 mg daily, and sublingual nitroglycerin as needed for chest pain.

Mr. Chen presents for routine follow-up and medication review. He reports chest discomfort 2-3 times per week, usually associated with climbing stairs or walking uphill. The discomfort typically resolves within 5 minutes of rest and responds well to one sublingual nitroglycerin tablet. He's been tracking his symptoms in a diary as instructed.

Current Assessment: Vital signs stable at Blood pressure 128/72, Heart rate 58, Respirations 16, Temperature 98.2°F. Physical examination reveals no acute distress, regular heart rhythm, clear lung sounds, and no peripheral edema. He appears well-informed about his condition but has questions about activity limitations and medication timing.

Patient Questions: "Should I take the nitroglycerin before I know I'll be active, like before climbing stairs? Sometimes I worry about exercising at all. How do I know if my chest pain is getting worse and I need to call the doctor?"

This scenario focuses on patient education and self-management skills for stable angina. The patient demonstrates good self-monitoring and appropriate use of sublingual nitroglycerin, but needs guidance on prophylactic medication use and symptom recognition that might indicate worsening condition.

Key cues include the predictable pattern of chest discomfort with exertion, appropriate response to rest and nitroglycerin, good medication adherence, and the patient's engagement in self-monitoring. The stable vital signs and controlled symptoms suggest his current management is effective.

NGN-Style Drag-and-Drop Question: Match each patient statement with the appropriate nursing response:

Patient Statements:

1. "Should I take nitroglycerin before activities that usually cause chest pain?"

2. "How do I know if my chest pain is getting worse?"

3. "Is it safe for me to exercise?"

Nursing Responses: A. "Call your doctor immediately if chest pain lasts more than 20 minutes, occurs at rest, or doesn't respond to two nitroglycerin tablets." B. "Yes, taking nitroglycerin 5 minutes before planned activity can prevent chest pain episodes." C. "Regular moderate exercise is beneficial, but start slowly and stop if you develop chest pain that doesn't resolve with rest."

Correct Matches: 1-B, 2-A, 3-C

Rationale: Prophylactic nitroglycerin use before activities known to trigger symptoms is an appropriate and recommended strategy for stable angina management. Teaching patients to recognize unstable angina patterns (prolonged duration, rest pain, poor response to medication) enables early recognition of potentially dangerous changes. Exercise counseling should balance the benefits of physical activity with appropriate precautions for patients with known coronary disease.

Scenario 4: Basic Heart Failure Management

Patient Presentation: Eleanor Washington, a 70-year-old retired librarian, presents to the outpatient heart failure clinic for routine follow-up. She has a history of heart failure with reduced ejection fraction (HFrEF) diagnosed eight months ago following a myocardial infarction. Her current medications include lisinopril 10 mg daily, metoprolol succinate 50 mg daily, furosemide 40 mg daily, and spironolactone 25 mg daily.

Mrs. Washington reports increased fatigue over the past week and notes that her wedding ring feels tighter than usual. Her home weight log shows: Monday 154 lbs, Tuesday 154 lbs, Wednesday 156 lbs, Thursday 157 lbs, Friday 159 lbs (today). Her baseline weight three weeks ago was 152 lbs. She denies chest pain but reports mild shortness of breath when climbing the stairs to her bedroom, which is new for her.

Physical Assessment: Alert and oriented, sitting comfortably at rest. Vital signs: Blood pressure 118/68, Heart rate 72, Respirations 20, Temperature 98.0°F, Oxygen saturation 94% on room air. Cardiovascular examination reveals regular rate and rhythm with an S3 gallop. Lung sounds reveal fine crackles at bilateral bases. Mild peripheral edema noted in ankles and feet bilaterally. Jugular venous distension estimated at 8 cm.

Laboratory Results: BNP 890 pg/mL (elevated from baseline of 420 pg/mL three months ago), creatinine 1.2 mg/dL (baseline 1.0 mg/dL), potassium 4.0 mEq/L, sodium 138 mEq/L.

This scenario focuses on recognizing early signs of heart failure exacerbation in a patient with established disease. The key learning objectives include identifying subtle changes that indicate fluid retention, understanding the significance of weight gain trends, and planning appropriate interventions for mild decompensation.

The constellation of findings—7-pound weight gain over five days, new dyspnea on exertion, physical signs of fluid retention (peripheral edema, JVD, crackles), and elevated BNP—suggests mild heart failure exacerbation requiring prompt intervention to prevent further deterioration.

NGN-Style Trend Analysis Question:

Review Mrs. Washington's weight trend and select the most appropriate interpretation:

Day 1: 154 lbs Day 2: 154 lbs
Day 3: 156 lbs (2 lb gain) Day 4: 157 lbs (3 lb gain from baseline) Day 5: 159 lbs (5 lb total gain from baseline)

A. Normal daily weight fluctuation requiring no intervention B. Gradual weight gain suggesting need for dietary counseling C. Concerning weight gain pattern indicating fluid retention and need for medication adjustment D. Expected weight gain following medication changes

Correct Answer: C

Rationale: A weight gain of 2-3 pounds over 2-3 days or 5 pounds in a week strongly suggests fluid retention in heart failure patients. This pattern, combined with her symptoms of increased fatigue and new dyspnea on exertion, indicates early decompensation requiring intervention. Heart failure patients should be taught to contact their healthcare provider for weight gains of this magnitude because early intervention can prevent hospitalization.

The trend shows acceleration in weight gain (stable for two days, then increasing daily), which is particularly concerning. Combined with her physical assessment findings of S3 gallop, crackles, peripheral edema, and elevated JVD, this represents clear evidence of fluid overload requiring diuretic adjustment.

Scenario 5: Peripheral Vascular Disease Assessment

Patient Presentation: Thomas Martinez, a 65-year-old retired construction worker, presents to the vascular clinic with complaints of leg cramping that occurs when he walks more than two blocks. The cramping consistently affects his left calf, starts after walking approximately the same distance, and resolves completely within 5 minutes of rest. He describes the pain as "tight and cramping, like a charley horse that won't let go."

Mr. Martinez has a 40-year smoking history (2 packs per day until quitting 5 years ago), diabetes mellitus type 2 for 15 years (HbA1c 7.8%), hypertension, and hyperlipidemia. His current medications include metformin 1000 mg twice daily, lisinopril 20 mg daily, atorvastatin 40 mg daily, and aspirin 81 mg daily.

Physical Assessment: Alert and cooperative, appears younger than stated age. Vital signs: Blood pressure 142/86, Heart rate 68, Respirations 16, Temperature 98.2°F. Cardiovascular examination reveals regular rate and rhythm, no murmurs. Pulmonary examination normal.

Lower extremity assessment reveals: Left leg appears slightly cooler than right, skin on left lower leg appears shiny with decreased hair growth, toenails thick and yellowish. Palpation of pulses: Right dorsalis pedis 2+, right posterior tibial 2+, left dorsalis pedis 1+, left posterior tibial barely palpable. Capillary refill on left foot 4 seconds (right foot 2 seconds). No open wounds or ulcerations noted.

Diagnostic Results: Ankle-brachial index (ABI): Right leg 0.95, Left leg 0.68 (abnormal, indicating significant arterial disease).

This scenario focuses on recognizing classic presentation of intermittent claudication and understanding the assessment techniques used to evaluate peripheral arterial disease. The patient's symptoms follow the typical pattern of claudication—predictable onset with activity, consistent location, and relief with rest.

Key assessment findings include the reduced pulses on the affected side, skin changes consistent with chronic ischemia, abnormal ABI indicating significant arterial stenosis, and the classic symptom pattern. The patient's risk factors (smoking history, diabetes, hypertension, hyperlipidemia) strongly support the diagnosis.

NGN-Style Bowtie Question:

Central Problem: 65-year-old male with intermittent claudication and abnormal ABI

Assessment Parameters (Select all that apply):

- Pedal pulse strength
- Capillary refill time
- Skin temperature
- Pain pattern with activity
- Ankle-brachial index
- Blood glucose levels
- Smoking history

Interventions (Select all that apply):

- Smoking cessation counseling

- Walking exercise program

- Foot care education

- Pain medication for claudication

- Immediate bed rest

- Surgical consultation referral

- Diabetes management optimization

Correct Selections: Assessment Parameters: Pedal pulse strength, capillary refill time, skin temperature, pain pattern with activity, ankle-brachial index **Interventions**: Smoking cessation counseling, walking exercise program, foot care education, surgical consultation referral, diabetes management optimization

Rationale: Assessment of peripheral arterial disease focuses on indicators of perfusion—pulse quality, capillary refill, skin temperature, and quantitative measures like ABI. While smoking history and diabetes are important risk factors, they're part of the history rather than ongoing assessment parameters.

Interventions for claudication include risk factor modification (smoking cessation, diabetes control), supervised exercise therapy (which paradoxically improves walking distance through collateral circulation development), and foot care education to prevent complications. Surgical consultation is appropriate for significant disease (ABI <0.70). Pain medications don't treat the underlying problem and bed rest would worsen the condition by further deconditioning the patient.

Chapter 7: Respiratory Scenarios

Scenario 6: COPD Stable Management

Patient Presentation: Harold Peterson, a 72-year-old retired mechanic, presents for routine follow-up of his moderate COPD. He was diagnosed 8 years ago and has been stable on his current regimen of tiotropium (Spiriva) 18 mcg daily via HandiHaler, albuterol MDI 2 puffs every 4-6 hours as needed, and home oxygen at 2 L/min continuous.

Mr. Peterson reports his usual morning cough with clear to white phlegm production, which he describes as "about the same as always." He can walk about 100 yards on level ground before needing to stop and rest. His oxygen saturation at rest on 2L oxygen is 92%. He quit smoking 3 years ago after a 45-year history of 1.5 packs per day.

Physical Assessment: Alert and oriented, speaking in full sentences at rest. Vital signs: Blood pressure 138/82, Heart rate 84, Respirations 22, Temperature 98.0°F, Oxygen saturation 92% on 2L nasal cannula. Pulmonary examination reveals decreased breath sounds bilaterally with expiratory wheeze, increased anteroposterior chest diameter (barrel chest), and use of accessory muscles for breathing.

Patient Education Needs: Mr. Peterson demonstrates correct use of his HandiHaler device but admits he sometimes forgets to rinse his mouth afterward. He's uncertain about when he should use his rescue inhaler and asks, "Should I use it before I get short of breath or wait until I really need it?"

This scenario focuses on stable COPD management, patient education needs, and recognizing normal baseline symptoms versus concerning changes. The patient demonstrates typical stable COPD presentation with characteristic physical findings and functional limitations.

Key teaching points include proper medication administration techniques, mouth rinsing after inhaled corticosteroids (though tiotropium is an anticholinergic, not a steroid, mouth rinsing is still recommended), and appropriate use of rescue medications.

NGN-Style Cloze Question:

Complete the patient education statement: "Mr. Peterson, you should use your albuterol rescue inhaler when you experience _____ or before activities that you know typically cause _____. After using your tiotropium HandiHaler, you should _____ to prevent _____. If you notice your sputum changing from clear or white to _____ or if you develop _____, you should contact your healthcare provider immediately."

Word Bank: increased shortness of breath, mouth infections, yellow or green, rinse your mouth with water, shortness of breath, fever

Correct Answers:

1. increased shortness of breath

2. shortness of breath

3. rinse your mouth with water

4. mouth infections

5. yellow or green

6. fever

Rationale: Rescue bronchodilators should be used for symptom relief or prophylactically before activities known to cause dyspnea. Mouth rinsing after inhaled medications helps prevent oral thrush and other mouth infections. Patients need to recognize signs of respiratory infection (purulent sputum, fever) that require prompt medical attention, as these can trigger COPD exacerbations.

Scenario 7: Community-Acquired Pneumonia

Patient Presentation: Maria Santos, a 58-year-old office manager, presents to the emergency department with a 3-day history of progressively worsening cough, fever, and shortness of breath. She initially thought she had a cold, but her symptoms have become more severe. She reports productive cough with yellow-green sputum, fever up to 101.5°F at home, and increasing difficulty with her usual activities due to shortness of breath.

Mrs. Santos has no significant past medical history and takes no regular medications. She denies smoking, recent travel, or sick contacts. She works in a well-ventilated office building and has not been hospitalized in over 10 years.

Physical Assessment: Appears mildly ill but alert and oriented. Vital signs: Blood pressure 118/72, Heart rate 102, Respirations 24, Temperature 101.2°F, Oxygen saturation 91% on room air. Pulmonary examination reveals decreased breath sounds and dullness to percussion over the right lower lobe, with inspiratory crackles noted in the same area. The remainder of her physical examination is normal.

Diagnostic Results: Chest X-ray shows right lower lobe consolidation consistent with pneumonia. White blood cell count 14,500/µL (elevated), with 82% neutrophils. Blood cultures drawn, awaiting results.

Treatment Plan: Admit for IV antibiotic therapy with ceftriaxone 1g daily and azithromycin 500mg daily, oxygen therapy to maintain saturation >92%, supportive care with fluids and symptomatic treatment.

This scenario focuses on recognizing typical presentation of community-acquired pneumonia and understanding the nursing care priorities for a patient with moderate illness requiring hospitalization.

NGN-Style Matrix Question:

Prioritize the following nursing interventions for Mrs. Santos:

Intervention	Priority Level
Administer prescribed antibiotics	High
Monitor oxygen saturation	High
Encourage fluid intake	Moderate
Obtain sputum culture	Moderate
Provide cough suppression	Low
Pain assessment	Moderate
Patient education about pneumonia	Low

Rationale: Antibiotic administration and oxygen monitoring represent high priorities because they directly address the infection and prevent respiratory compromise. Fluid intake and sputum culture collection are important but not immediately life-threatening. Cough suppression is generally not recommended in pneumonia as coughing helps clear infected secretions. Patient education, while important, can be deferred until the acute phase is stabilized.

Scenario 8: Asthma Action Plan Implementation

Patient Presentation: Jennifer Walsh, a 45-year-old high school teacher, comes to the clinic for routine asthma follow-up. She has mild persistent asthma controlled with fluticasone/salmeterol (Advair) 100/50 twice daily and albuterol MDI as needed for rescue. She reports good control most of the time but has questions about managing her asthma during the upcoming spring allergy season.

Ms. Walsh monitors her peak flow daily and brings her peak flow diary showing readings that range from 380-420 L/min (her personal best is 420 L/min). She reports using her rescue inhaler 1-2 times per week, usually in association with cleaning her classroom or exposure to strong perfumes.

Current Assessment: Alert and comfortable, no acute distress. Vital signs: Blood pressure 122/78, Heart rate 72, Respirations 16, Temperature 98.4°F, Oxygen saturation 98% on room air. Pulmonary examination reveals clear breath sounds bilaterally, no wheeze or prolonged expiration noted. Current peak flow measurement is 410 L/min.

Patient Questions: "I know spring is coming and my allergies usually get worse. Should I increase my medicine before I start having problems? What should I do if my peak flow starts dropping? When should I worry and call the doctor?"

This scenario focuses on asthma self-management education and helping patients understand how to use their asthma action plan effectively. The patient demonstrates good baseline control but needs guidance on managing seasonal variations and recognizing when her condition is worsening.

NGN-Style Drag-and-Drop Sequencing:

Arrange the following actions in the order Ms. Walsh should take if her peak flow drops to 320 L/min (76% of personal best):

Available Actions:

- Contact healthcare provider
- Use rescue inhaler
- Rest and avoid triggers
- Measure peak flow again in 20 minutes
- Consider oral prednisone if prescribed
- Continue daily controller medication

Correct Sequence:

1. Use rescue inhaler
2. Rest and avoid triggers

3. Continue daily controller medication

4. Measure peak flow again in 20 minutes

5. Contact healthcare provider

6. Consider oral prednisone if prescribed

Rationale: Peak flow of 76% of personal best indicates the "yellow zone" of asthma management, requiring immediate bronchodilator use followed by reassessment. If peak flow doesn't improve to the green zone (>80% personal best) after rescue medication, medical consultation is needed. Oral corticosteroids might be prescribed for yellow zone episodes that don't respond adequately to bronchodilators. Controller medications should be continued during exacerbations unless specifically contraindicated.

Scenario 9: Post-Operative Breathing Exercises

Patient Presentation: William Chen, a 60-year-old accountant, is 24 hours post-operative following elective laparoscopic cholecystectomy. His surgery was uncomplicated, lasting 90 minutes, and he recovered normally from general anesthesia. He has been ambulating with assistance and tolerating clear liquids.

Mr. Chen reports incisional pain rated 4/10 (managed with acetaminophen and tramadol), but he's reluctant to cough or take deep breaths because it increases his discomfort. He's concerned about "hurting something inside" if he coughs too forcefully. His incentive spirometer readings have been consistently low, achieving only 1000 mL when his predicted volume should be 2500 mL.

Physical Assessment: Alert and oriented, ambulatory with minimal assistance. Vital signs: Blood pressure 132/84, Heart rate 88, Respirations 20, Temperature 98.8°F, Oxygen saturation 94% on room air. Pulmonary examination reveals diminished breath sounds at bilateral bases with fine crackles noted. No signs of respiratory distress at rest.

Risk Factors: Age 60, abdominal surgery, general anesthesia, reluctance to cough due to pain, decreased mobility initially post-operative.

This scenario focuses on preventing post-operative pulmonary complications through effective patient education and pain management strategies that enable participation in respiratory exercises.

NGN-Style Highlighting Question:

Highlight the assessment findings that indicate risk for pulmonary complications:

"Mr. Chen is 24 hours post-operative following laparoscopic cholecystectomy under general anesthesia. He reports incisional pain rated 4/10 and is reluctant to cough or take deep breaths due to discomfort. His incentive spirometer volumes are 1000 mL compared to predicted 2500 mL. Physical examination reveals diminished breath sounds at bilateral bases with fine crackles. Oxygen saturation is 94% on room air, and he's been ambulatory with assistance."

Items to Highlight:

- reluctant to cough or take deep breaths due to discomfort

- incentive spirometer volumes are 1000 mL compared to predicted 2500 mL

- diminished breath sounds at bilateral bases with fine crackles

- Oxygen saturation is 94% on room air

Rationale: These findings suggest developing atelectasis and risk for pneumonia. Reluctance to breathe deeply due to pain leads to decreased lung expansion, evidenced by poor incentive spirometry performance and physical findings of diminished breath sounds and crackles. The oxygen saturation of 94%, while not critically low, represents decreased oxygenation that could worsen without intervention.

Scenario 10: Sleep Apnea Management

Patient Presentation: Robert Johnson, a 52-year-old truck driver, presents for follow-up after being diagnosed with moderate obstructive sleep apnea following a sleep study. His Apnea-Hypopnea Index (AHI) was 22 events per hour. He's been prescribed CPAP therapy at 8 cm H2O pressure and has been using it for two weeks.

Mr. Johnson reports difficulty adjusting to the CPAP machine, stating "I feel like I'm suffocating with that thing on my face. I end up taking it off in the middle of the night." He's been able to use it for only 3-4 hours per night on average. His wife reports that his snoring has decreased when he uses the machine, but he still seems tired during the day.

Current Assessment: Alert but appears fatigued. BMI 34 (obese). Vital signs: Blood pressure 142/88, Heart rate 78, Respirations 16, Temperature 98.2°F, Oxygen saturation 96% on room air. Physical examination reveals large neck circumference (18 inches), crowded oropharynx, and no acute distress.

CPAP Data Download: Shows average usage of 3.2 hours per night, mask leak rate elevated at 15 L/min, AHI on CPAP therapy reduced to 8 events per hour when machine is used.

This scenario focuses on CPAP therapy adherence challenges and problem-solving strategies to improve treatment compliance for sleep apnea.

NGN-Style Multiple Response Question:

Select all appropriate interventions to improve Mr. Johnson's CPAP adherence:

A. Recommend discontinuing CPAP therapy due to poor tolerance B. Suggest trying a different mask style or size C. Gradual acclimatization starting with short daytime periods D. Address mask leak issues with equipment adjustment E. Provide reassurance that discomfort will resolve in 1-2 days F. Discuss the health consequences of untreated sleep apnea G. Consider referral to sleep medicine specialist for therapy adjustment

Correct Answers: B, C, D, F, G

Rationale: CPAP adherence challenges are common and usually addressable through equipment adjustments, gradual acclimatization, patient education, and professional support. Different mask styles may provide better comfort and seal. Gradual acclimatization helps patients adjust to the sensation. Addressing mask leaks improves comfort and therapy effectiveness. Education about health consequences motivates adherence. Sleep specialist referral may be needed for therapy optimization. Discontinuing therapy isn't appropriate for moderate sleep apnea, and discomfort typically takes weeks, not days, to resolve.

Key Learning Points

- Beginner scenarios focus on single-system problems with clear presentations and established protocols

- Pattern recognition skills develop through repeated exposure to similar clinical situations with systematic analysis

- Effective cue recognition requires distinguishing between normal findings and significant changes requiring intervention

- Patient education represents a crucial nursing intervention that requires understanding both the medical condition and adult learning principles

- Medication management involves not just administration but understanding indications, contraindications, and patient teaching needs

- Risk factor identification helps predict potential complications and guide preventive interventions

- Assessment skills must be systematic and focused on findings relevant to the patient's primary condition

- Pain management requires balancing comfort with functional goals, particularly in post-operative patients

- Adherence challenges are common with chronic disease management and require individualized problem-solving approaches

- Documentation of trends (weights, peak flows, symptoms) provides crucial information for ongoing care management

Chapter 8: Gastrointestinal Scenarios

The heart beats roughly 100,000 times each day, pumping life through every vessel and capillary in the human body. For nursing students, cardiovascular conditions represent some of the most common yet potentially challenging situations you'll encounter in clinical practice. These five foundational scenarios guide you through essential cardiovascular nursing skills—from managing stable hypertension to recognizing post-procedure complications.

Scenario 11: Peptic Ulcer Disease Management

Patient Background: James Mitchell, a 48-year-old insurance broker, arrives at the outpatient clinic for follow-up after being diagnosed with H. pylori-positive peptic ulcer disease six weeks ago. He completed his initial triple therapy regimen (clarithromycin, amoxicillin, and omeprazole) two weeks ago and returns for symptom assessment and treatment evaluation.

Mr. Mitchell originally presented with epigastric pain that worsened after eating, particularly spicy or acidic foods. The pain felt like "burning" and often woke him at night around 2-3 AM. His H. pylori breath test came back positive, and upper endoscopy revealed a 1.2 cm duodenal ulcer with no signs of bleeding or perforation.

His medical history includes mild hypertension controlled with lisinopril 10 mg daily and occasional tension headaches. He drinks 2-3 cups of coffee daily, rarely consumes alcohol, and quit smoking five years ago after a 20-year habit. He works long hours and admits to irregular eating patterns, often skipping breakfast and eating large dinners late in the evening (13).

Current Assessment: Mr. Mitchell appears comfortable and reports significant improvement in his symptoms. "The burning pain is almost completely gone," he states. "I can eat pizza again without doubling over afterward." He's been taking omeprazole 40 mg daily as prescribed and hasn't needed any antacids for the past week.

His vital signs show blood pressure 128/82, heart rate 72, respirations 16, and temperature 98.4°F. Physical examination reveals a soft, non-tender abdomen with normal bowel sounds. No guarding or rebound tenderness is present. He weighs 175 pounds, which represents a 3-pound weight gain since his initial diagnosis (he had lost weight due to decreased appetite from pain).

Laboratory Results: Complete blood count shows hemoglobin 13.8 g/dL (improved from 12.1 g/dL at diagnosis), hematocrit 41%, and white blood cell count 6,200/μL. His iron levels have returned to normal range. H. pylori stool antigen test scheduled for next week to confirm eradication.

NGN-Style Cloze Question: Complete the patient education statement for Mr. Mitchell:

"Mr. Mitchell, now that you've completed your antibiotic treatment, you should continue taking _____ for at least _____ more weeks to allow complete ulcer healing. You can gradually reintroduce _____ foods, but avoid _____ and _____ which can delay healing. If you experience any return of _____, _____, or _____, contact our office immediately. We'll check your _____ test next week to confirm the bacteria is gone."

Answer Choices: omeprazole, 4-6, acidic or spicy, NSAIDs, alcohol, burning pain, nausea, black stools, H. pylori stool antigen

Correct Completion: omeprazole, 4-6, acidic or spicy, NSAIDs, alcohol, burning pain, nausea, black stools, H. pylori stool antigen

Clinical Reasoning: PPI therapy continues for 4-8 weeks after antibiotic completion to ensure ulcer healing. NSAIDs can impair healing and increase bleeding risk. Black stools indicate possible GI bleeding requiring immediate evaluation. H. pylori testing confirms bacterial eradication, typically done 4 weeks after antibiotic completion (14).

Scenario 12: Constipation in Elderly Patient

Patient Background: Dorothy Chen, a 78-year-old retired librarian, presents to her primary care provider with concerns about changes in her bowel habits over the past three months. She reports having bowel movements only every 3-4 days compared to her usual daily pattern. The stools are hard, requiring significant straining, and she feels incompletely evacuated afterward.

Mrs. Chen lives independently in a senior apartment complex. Her medical history includes osteoarthritis (managed with acetaminophen and occasional ibuprofen), mild cognitive impairment, and seasonal allergies. Her medications include alendronate weekly, calcium with vitamin D daily, multivitamin, and diphenhydramine as needed for sleep.

She describes her typical daily routine: She wakes around 6 AM, has coffee and toast for breakfast, watches morning television programs, and takes short walks in the building's hallways. Her fluid intake consists mainly of coffee (3-4 cups daily) and one glass of water with meals. She eats smaller portions than previously due to decreased appetite and concern about food costs (15).

Current Assessment: Mrs. Chen appears well-groomed but moves slowly due to arthritis stiffness. Her vital signs show blood pressure 142/88, heart rate 68, respirations 18, and temperature 98.2°F. Abdominal examination reveals mild distension with palpable stool in the left lower quadrant. Bowel sounds are present but hypoactive. Digital rectal examination shows hard stool in the rectal vault.

She reports no abdominal pain but describes feeling "bloated and uncomfortable." Her last bowel movement was four days ago, requiring 20 minutes of straining and produced small, hard pellets. She's tried increasing her fiber intake by eating more bread and crackers but hasn't noticed improvement.

Bowel Pattern Analysis:

- Week 1: Bowel movements on days 1, 4, 7 (every 2-3 days)

- Week 2: Bowel movements on days 3, 6 (every 3 days)

- Week 3: Bowel movements on days 2, 6 (every 4 days)

- Week 4: Bowel movements on days 1, 5 (every 4 days)

NGN-Style Trend Analysis: Review Mrs. Chen's bowel pattern trend and select the most appropriate nursing intervention priority:

The pattern shows progressively decreasing frequency from every 2-3 days to every 4 days, with increasing difficulty and incomplete evacuation. This trend indicates:

A. Normal age-related changes requiring no intervention B. Acute constipation requiring immediate laxative therapy C. Chronic constipation requiring multifaceted intervention approach D. Possible bowel obstruction requiring emergency evaluation

Correct Answer: C

Rationale: The gradual worsening over three months with incomplete evacuation and straining indicates chronic functional constipation common in elderly patients. Multiple factors contribute including medications (diphenhydramine), decreased mobility, inadequate fluid intake, and possibly inadequate fiber. Management requires addressing multiple causes rather than just symptom treatment (16).

Intervention Plan: Discontinue diphenhydramine (anticholinergic effects worsen constipation), increase water intake to 6-8 glasses daily, add soluble fiber sources like oatmeal and fruits, encourage regular walking, establish consistent bathroom routine after meals, and consider gentle laxatives if lifestyle modifications insufficient.

Scenario 13: GERD Lifestyle Modifications

Patient Background: Michael Rodriguez, a 55-year-old high school principal, seeks help for worsening heartburn and regurgitation symptoms that have been affecting his sleep and daily activities for the past six months. He describes a burning sensation in his chest that occurs 3-4 times weekly, usually in the evening after dinner and sometimes during the night when lying flat.

Mr. Rodriguez's symptoms started gradually but have intensified recently. He notices the burning is worse after eating tomato-based foods, citrus fruits, coffee, and chocolate. Large meals consistently trigger symptoms, and he's started avoiding his favorite Mexican and Italian restaurants. The symptoms wake him around 2-3 AM, forcing him to sleep in his recliner chair to find relief.

His work stress has increased this academic year due to budget cuts and staff reductions. He often eats lunch quickly at his desk and has dinner late (around 8-9 PM) after attending evening school events. His weight has increased 15 pounds over the past two years, bringing his BMI to 29. He drinks 4-5 cups of coffee daily and occasionally has wine with dinner on weekends (17).

Current Assessment: Mr. Rodriguez appears tired but alert. Vital signs show blood pressure 138/86, heart rate 76, respirations 16, and temperature 98.6°F. Physical examination reveals mild epigastric tenderness and a slightly distended abdomen. No alarming symptoms like difficulty swallowing, weight loss, or blood in stool are present.

He reports that antacids provide temporary relief (30-60 minutes) but symptoms return. He's been taking over-the-counter ranitidine occasionally but finds limited benefit. His sleep quality has deteriorated, affecting his concentration and energy during work hours.

Symptom Trigger Analysis:

- **Food triggers**: Tomato sauce, citrus fruits, chocolate, coffee, spicy foods, large meals

- **Timing patterns**: Symptoms worse in evening, especially after 6 PM meals

- **Positional factors**: Lying flat worsens symptoms, upright position provides relief

- **Lifestyle factors**: Stress, late eating, quick meals, weight gain

NGN-Style Matrix for Symptom Triggers:

Categorize the following factors as "Major Trigger," "Minor Trigger," or "Not a Trigger" for Mr. Rodriguez's GERD symptoms:

Foods and Habits Assessment:

- Tomato-based sauces: Major Trigger
- Coffee consumption: Major Trigger
- Large meal portions: Major Trigger
- Eating close to bedtime: Major Trigger
- Chocolate consumption: Minor Trigger
- Weekend wine: Minor Trigger
- Work stress: Minor Trigger
- Morning toast: Not a Trigger

Rationale: Major triggers directly correlate with symptom onset and severity. Acidic foods (tomatoes, citrus), caffeine, large meals, and eating within 3 hours of bedtime consistently worsen GERD symptoms. Weight gain and lying flat after meals increase intra-abdominal pressure and promote reflux (18).

Comprehensive Management Plan:

1. **Dietary modifications**: Eliminate trigger foods for 2-4 weeks, reduce meal portions, avoid eating within 3 hours of bedtime

2. **Lifestyle changes**: Elevate head of bed 6-8 inches, lose 10-15 pounds, reduce coffee to 1-2 cups daily

3. **Stress management**: Regular exercise, relaxation techniques, consistent meal timing

4. **Medical evaluation**: Trial PPI therapy, consider upper endoscopy if symptoms persis

Chapter 9: Endocrine Scenarios

Scenario 14: Type 2 Diabetes Routine Management

Patient Background: Patricia Williams, a 60-year-old retired nurse, comes for her quarterly diabetes management appointment. She was diagnosed with Type 2 diabetes mellitus four years ago and has been managing her condition with metformin 1000 mg twice daily and lifestyle modifications. Her most recent HbA1c three months ago was 7.2%.

Mrs. Williams checks her blood glucose twice daily using a glucometer and maintains a detailed log. She follows a diabetic diet plan developed with a nutritionist, limiting carbohydrates to 45-60 grams per meal. She walks 30 minutes most days and attends a senior fitness class twice weekly at her community center.

Recent concerns include occasional episodes of dizziness in the late afternoon and difficulty maintaining her target weight. She's gained 5 pounds over the past six months despite following her diet plan. Her blood pressure has also been trending upward, with home readings averaging 145/88 over the past month (19).

Current Assessment: Mrs. Williams appears well and engaged in her care. Her vital signs show blood pressure 148/90, heart rate 72, respirations 16, temperature 98.4°F, and weight 168 pounds (up from 163 pounds six months ago). Physical examination reveals no acute abnormalities. Her feet show good sensation and circulation with no lesions or calluses.

Blood Glucose Log Analysis (Past 2 Weeks):

- **Morning readings**: Range 110-145 mg/dL, average 128 mg/dL

- **Evening readings**: Range 125-165 mg/dL, average 142 mg/dL

- **Pattern observations**: Higher readings on weekends, lowest readings on exercise days

- **Hypoglycemic episodes**: None recorded, but reports occasional dizziness around 4 PM

Laboratory Results: HbA1c 7.8% (increased from 7.2%), fasting glucose 135 mg/dL, creatinine 0.9 mg/dL, microalbumin/creatinine ratio 25 mg/g (normal <30), lipid panel shows total cholesterol 195 mg/dL, LDL 118 mg/dL.

NGN-Style Trend Analysis:

Review Mrs. Williams' glucose pattern trends and HbA1c progression:

Three-Month Comparison:

- Previous HbA1c: 7.2%

- Current HbA1c: 7.8%

- Average morning glucose: Increased from 115 mg/dL to 128 mg/dL

- Average evening glucose: Increased from 130 mg/dL to 142 mg/dL

- Weight change: +5 pounds

This trend indicates:

A. Well-controlled diabetes with normal progression B. Worsening glycemic control requiring medication adjustment C. Acute diabetic emergency requiring immediate intervention D. Hypoglycemia risk requiring medication reduction

Correct Answer: B

Rationale: The HbA1c increase from 7.2% to 7.8% indicates worsening long-term glucose control. Both fasting and postprandial glucose levels have increased despite continued lifestyle adherence. Weight gain may contribute to insulin resistance. The American Diabetes Association target HbA1c is <7% for most adults, making medication intensification appropriate (20).

Management Adjustments:

73

1. **Medication**: Consider adding second agent (sulfonylurea, DPP-4 inhibitor, or SGLT-2 inhibitor)

2. **Lifestyle review**: Reassess portion sizes, weekend eating patterns, exercise intensity

3. **Monitoring**: Increase glucose checks to include 2-hour post-meal readings

4. **Blood pressure**: Initiate ACE inhibitor given diabetes and hypertension

5. **Education**: Review sick-day management, hypoglycemia recognition

Scenario 15: Hypothyroidism Medication Management

Patient Background: Linda Thompson, a 45-year-old marketing executive, presents for follow-up six weeks after starting levothyroxine 50 mcg daily for newly diagnosed hypothyroidism. She was diagnosed following complaints of fatigue, weight gain, cold intolerance, and difficulty concentrating that had been worsening over the past year.

Her initial thyroid function tests showed TSH 12.8 mU/L (normal 0.4-4.0) and free T4 0.7 ng/dL (normal 0.8-1.8). She has no family history of thyroid disease and no history of neck radiation or thyroid surgery. Her symptoms had significantly impacted her work performance and personal relationships.

Ms. Thompson reports some improvement in her energy levels since starting medication but still feels "not quite right." She's been taking her levothyroxine every morning on an empty stomach, waiting at least 30 minutes before eating as instructed. She hasn't missed any doses and stores the medication in a cool, dry place away from her other supplements (21).

Current Assessment: Ms. Thompson appears more alert than her previous visit but still reports feeling tired by mid-afternoon. Her vital signs show blood pressure 118/76, heart rate 68, respirations 16, and temperature 98.2°F. She's lost 3 pounds since starting treatment. Her reflexes appear brisker than previously noted.

Symptom Improvement Assessment:

- **Energy levels**: Improved from "exhausted all day" to "tired by afternoon"

- **Cold intolerance**: Still present but less severe

- **Weight**: Lost 3 pounds (was gaining 1-2 pounds monthly before treatment)

- **Concentration**: Some improvement in mental clarity

- **Sleep quality**: Slightly better, but still not refreshing

- **Hair and skin**: No change noted yet (takes 3-6 months)

Laboratory Results: TSH 8.2 mU/L (decreased from 12.8), free T4 1.0 ng/dL (improved from 0.7). These results indicate partial response to treatment but suggest need for dose adjustment.

NGN-Style Highlighting Question:

Highlight the assessment findings that indicate need for levothyroxine dose adjustment:

"Ms. Thompson reports improved energy levels since starting levothyroxine 50 mcg daily six weeks ago. Her TSH decreased from 12.8 to 8.2 mU/L, and free T4 increased from 0.7 to 1.0 ng/dL. She's lost 3 pounds and feels more alert, but still experiences afternoon fatigue and cold intolerance. She takes her medication correctly on an empty stomach every morning and hasn't missed doses. Her heart rate remains 68 bpm, and reflexes are brisker than baseline."

Items to Highlight:

- TSH decreased from 12.8 to 8.2 mU/L (still elevated above normal range)

- still experiences afternoon fatigue and cold intolerance

- Her heart rate remains 68 bpm (bradycardia persists)

Rationale: TSH of 8.2 mU/L remains well above the normal range (0.4-4.0), indicating inadequate thyroid hormone replacement. Persistent symptoms of fatigue and cold intolerance, along with continued bradycardia, suggest clinical hypothyroidism despite treatment. Dose increase is typically needed when TSH remains above 4.0 mU/L after 6-8 weeks of therapy (22).

Medication Adjustment Plan:

1. **Dose increase**: Levothyroxine increased to 75 mcg daily

2. **Monitoring**: Recheck TSH and free T4 in 6-8 weeks

3. **Target goals**: TSH 0.4-2.5 mU/L, symptom resolution

4. **Patient education**: Expected timeline for symptom improvement (2-4 months for full effect)

5. **Drug interactions**: Review for medications affecting absorption (iron, calcium, coffee)

Scenario 16: Diabetic Foot Care Education

Patient Background: Robert Martinez, a 65-year-old retired construction worker, attends a diabetes education session focused on foot care. He's had Type 2 diabetes for 12 years with generally good control (HbA1c 7.1%) but has developed peripheral neuropathy over the past three years. He reports decreased sensation in both feet, particularly the toes, and occasional cramping in his calves during walking.

Mr. Martinez lives with his wife in a single-story home and remains active with yard work and home maintenance projects. He typically wears work boots during outside activities and goes barefoot inside the house. His vision is good with reading glasses, and he can reach his feet adequately for self-care.

His diabetes complications include mild retinopathy (stable, monitored annually) and the peripheral neuropathy. His current medications include metformin 1000 mg twice daily, glimepiride 4 mg daily, and atorvastatin 20 mg daily. Blood pressure is well-controlled with lisinopril (23).

Current Assessment: Mr. Martinez's feet show signs of chronic diabetes effects. Both feet have decreased hair growth and slightly shiny, thin skin. Pedal pulses are palpable but diminished. Monofilament testing reveals decreased sensation in all toes and the plantar surface of both feet. No open wounds, calluses, or deformities are present.

His toenails are thick and yellowish but properly trimmed. He demonstrates difficulty distinguishing between sharp and dull sensation when tested with a safety pin. Capillary refill in his toes is 4 seconds (normal <3 seconds), indicating mild circulatory compromise.

Risk Assessment Findings:

- **Neuropathy**: Loss of protective sensation in both feet
- **Vascular status**: Diminished but present pulses, delayed capillary refill
- **Skin condition**: Dry, thin skin prone to breakdown
- **Nail condition**: Thickened nails requiring careful trimming
- **Vision and mobility**: Adequate for self-care activities
- **Knowledge level**: Limited understanding of diabetic foot risks

NGN-Style Drag-and-Drop for Foot Care Steps:

Arrange the following daily diabetic foot care steps in the correct sequence:

Available Steps:

- Apply moisturizer to feet (avoiding between toes)

- Inspect feet for cuts, blisters, or changes
- Wash feet with warm (not hot) water and mild soap
- Dry feet thoroughly, especially between toes
- Put on clean, dry socks
- Test water temperature with elbow or thermometer
- Choose appropriate footwear for the day's activities

Correct Sequence:

1. Test water temperature with elbow or thermometer
2. Wash feet with warm (not hot) water and mild soap
3. Dry feet thoroughly, especially between toes
4. Inspect feet for cuts, blisters, or changes
5. Apply moisturizer to feet (avoiding between toes)
6. Put on clean, dry socks
7. Choose appropriate footwear for the day's activities

Rationale: This sequence ensures safety (temperature testing prevents burns), cleanliness, thorough inspection when feet are clean and dry, proper moisturization without creating fungal growth conditions, and appropriate protection. Daily inspection is crucial for early detection of problems in patients with decreased sensation (24).

Comprehensive Education Plan:

Daily foot care routine: Temperature testing, gentle washing, thorough drying, daily inspection with mirror if needed, moisturizing (not between toes), clean socks, proper footwear selection.

Risk reduction strategies: Never go barefoot (even indoors), inspect shoes for foreign objects before wearing, trim nails straight across, avoid tight socks or shoes, protect feet from temperature extremes.

When to seek help: Any cut, blister, redness, swelling, drainage, ingrown nail, or change in skin color. Patients with neuropathy should have professional foot care for calluses or nail problems.

Professional care schedule: Podiatry visits every 3-6 months for nail care and foot health assessment, immediate evaluation for any concerning changes, annual comprehensive foot screening by healthcare provider.

Clinical Reasoning Summary

These beginner gastrointestinal and endocrine scenarios build foundational assessment and management skills for common chronic conditions. Each scenario emphasizes patient education, symptom monitoring, and recognition of when conditions require intervention or specialist referral.

The progression from peptic ulcer management through diabetic foot care demonstrates increasing complexity in patient education needs and self-management skills. Students learn to recognize normal healing patterns, identify concerning changes, and provide education that prevents complications.

Key assessment skills developed: Symptom pattern recognition, medication adherence evaluation, lifestyle factor analysis, patient education effectiveness, and appropriate timing for follow-up or specialist referral.

Clinical reasoning progression: Students move from identifying obvious problems (active peptic ulcer symptoms) to recognizing subtle changes requiring intervention (TSH levels indicating medication adjustment needs) to preventing future complications (diabetic foot care education).

Closing Observations

The beauty of these foundational scenarios lies not in their complexity, but in their ability to build systematic thinking patterns that serve nurses throughout their careers. Each patient teaches us something different about the intersection between pathophysiology and human experience—how Mr. Mitchell's work stress influences his eating patterns, how Mrs. Chen's independence affects her willingness to discuss bathroom habits, or how Mr. Martinez's construction background shapes his approach to foot care.

These scenarios remind us that nursing's strength comes from understanding both the science behind the conditions and the individual human factors that influence each patient's experience. The protocols and procedures matter, but the real skill lies in adapting those guidelines to meet each person's unique needs and circumstances.

Key Learning Points

- Patient education requires understanding both medical conditions and individual learning needs

- Chronic disease management focuses on symptom monitoring and preventing complications

- Medication management involves dosing, timing, adherence, and recognition of therapeutic effectiveness

- Lifestyle modifications require individualized approaches based on patient capabilities and preferences

- Assessment skills must distinguish between normal healing patterns and concerning changes

- Risk factor identification guides both immediate care and long-term prevention strategies

- Documentation of symptom patterns provides crucial information for ongoing care decisions

- Patient self-management skills require ongoing reinforcement and adaptation over time

- Professional collaboration ensures comprehensive care for complex chronic conditions

- Early intervention prevents complications and improves long-term outcomes

Chapter 10: Basic Safety and Comfort Scenarios

Patient safety forms the bedrock of nursing practice—every intervention, assessment, and decision you make carries the potential to either protect or harm the individuals in your care. These four scenarios address fundamental safety concerns that transcend specific medical diagnoses: fall prevention, pressure injury prevention, pain management, and medication safety. Each situation requires you to think systematically about risk factors while maintaining focus on patient comfort and dignity.

Scenario 17: Fall Risk Assessment and Prevention

Patient Background: Eleanor Washington, a 75-year-old retired elementary school teacher, was admitted to the medical unit three days ago following a fall at home that resulted in a minor head injury and left wrist fracture. She lives alone in a two-story colonial home where she's resided for 40 years, and this fall occurred when she was coming downstairs to answer the telephone around 10 PM.

Mrs. Washington describes the incident as "losing my footing" on the carpeted stairs. She doesn't recall exactly what happened but remembers sitting at the bottom of the stairs with a headache and wrist pain. A neighbor found her the next morning when she didn't pick up her newspaper as usual. Her CT scan showed no intracranial bleeding, and her wrist fracture was treated with a cast.

Her medical history includes mild osteoporosis, hypertension controlled with hydrochlorothiazide 25 mg daily, and recent initiation of zolpidem 5 mg for sleep difficulties. She wears bifocal glasses and uses a magnifying glass for reading small print. Her daughter lives two hours away and visits monthly (25).

Current Assessment: Mrs. Washington is alert and oriented but appears somewhat unsteady when ambulating. Her vital signs are stable at blood pressure 128/78, heart rate 72, respirations 16, and temperature 98.4°F. She moves cautiously, favoring her casted left

82

arm, and asks for assistance when getting out of bed despite being cleared for independent ambulation.

Fall Risk Assessment Using Morse Fall Scale:

- **History of falling**: Yes, recent fall = 25 points
- **Secondary diagnosis**: Wrist fracture, mild head injury = 15 points
- **Ambulatory aid**: None currently, but unsteady gait = 15 points
- **IV/heparin lock**: No = 0 points
- **Gait**: Weak, unsteady = 20 points
- **Mental status**: Alert, oriented = 0 points
- **Total Score**: 75 points (High risk: >51 points)

Environmental and Personal Risk Factors:

- **Medication effects**: Zolpidem increases fall risk, hydrochlorothiazide may cause orthostatic hypotension
- **Visual impairment**: Bifocals can affect depth perception, especially on stairs
- **Home environment**: Two-story home with stairs, loose carpeting potential
- **Age-related changes**: Decreased muscle strength, slower reflexes, balance changes
- **Recent trauma**: Confidence affected by recent fall experience

NGN-Style Bowtie for Fall Prevention:

Central Problem: 75-year-old with high fall risk (Morse score 75) and recent fall history

Assessment Parameters (Select all that apply):

- Orthostatic vital signs

- Gait stability and balance

- Medication review for fall risk drugs

- Vision assessment with current glasses

- Cognitive assessment for judgment

- Muscle strength evaluation

- Environmental hazard identification

Interventions (Select all that apply):

- Place bed in lowest position with brakes locked

- Ensure call light within reach at all times

- Provide non-slip socks or shoes for ambulation

- Remove scatter rugs and unnecessary furniture

- Install grab bars in bathroom areas

- Review medications with physician for alternatives

- Provide bedside commode for nighttime use

- Educate patient about fall risk factors

Correct Selections: Assessment Parameters: All listed items are appropriate for comprehensive fall risk assessment **Interventions**: All listed interventions are evidence-based fall prevention strategies

Rationale: Comprehensive fall risk assessment examines multiple factors including medications, vision, cognition, strength, and environmental hazards. Evidence-based interventions address modifiable risk factors while maintaining patient independence and dignity. The goal is risk reduction, not elimination of all activity (26).

Case Development: During Mrs. Washington's hospitalization, staff implements a comprehensive fall prevention plan. Her zolpidem is discontinued and replaced with sleep hygiene education. Physical therapy evaluates her gait and provides a walker for added stability.

Occupational therapy assesses her home environment and recommends modifications including stair railings, bathroom grab bars, and improved lighting.

The nursing staff ensures her call light is always within reach, provides non-slip socks, and maintains her bed in the lowest position. They teach her to sit on the bedside for 30 seconds before standing and to use the bathroom before bedtime to reduce nighttime trips.

Discharge Planning Considerations: Home safety evaluation, family education about fall prevention, follow-up with primary care provider for medication review, physical therapy referral for strength and balance training, and discussion about home modifications or alternative living arrangements if needed.

Scenario 18: Pressure Injury Prevention

Patient Background: Harold Peterson, an 82-year-old retired farmer, was admitted to the medical unit five days ago with pneumonia and dehydration. His condition has stabilized, but he remains weak and spends most of his time in bed or sitting in a chair. He has lost 15 pounds over the past month due to poor appetite and difficulty preparing meals at home.

Mr. Peterson lives alone on his farm since his wife died two years ago. His son visits weekly but lives 50 miles away. He has diabetes mellitus (HbA1c 8.2%), peripheral vascular disease, and chronic kidney disease stage 3. His medications include metformin, lisinopril, and atorvastatin. He's been incontinent of urine intermittently since admission due to weakness and delayed response to urges (27).

Current Assessment: Mr. Peterson appears frail and moves slowly. His skin is dry and thin with decreased turgor. He weighs 145 pounds (down from 160 pounds baseline). Vital signs show blood pressure 110/68, heart rate 88, respirations 20, and temperature 98.6°F. He requires assistance with position changes and transfers.

Braden Scale Assessment:

- **Sensory perception**: Slightly limited (responds to verbal commands but cannot communicate discomfort) = 3 points

- **Moisture**: Occasionally moist (skin occasionally moist from incontinence) = 3 points

- **Activity**: Bedfast (confined to bed most of the time) = 1 point

- **Mobility**: Very limited (makes occasional slight position changes) = 2 points

- **Nutrition**: Probably inadequate (eating less than half of meals) = 2 points

- **Friction and shear**: Potential problem (moves feebly, requires assistance) = 2 points

- **Total Score**: 13 points (High risk: ≤18 points)

Current Skin Assessment:

- **Coccyx area**: Stage 1 pressure injury with non-blanchable redness

- **Both heels**: Redness that blanches with pressure relief

- **Left hip**: Small area of skin breakdown from lying on side

- **Sacrum**: Intact but reddened after prolonged sitting

- **Overall condition**: Dry, fragile skin with poor elasticity

NGN-Style Matrix for Risk Factors:

Categorize the following factors as "High Risk," "Moderate Risk," or "Low Risk" for pressure injury development:

Patient Factors Assessment:

- Advanced age (82 years): High Risk

- Diabetes with poor control: High Risk

- Immobility and bedrest: High Risk

- Incontinence episodes: High Risk

- Significant weight loss: High Risk

- Peripheral vascular disease: Moderate Risk

- Chronic kidney disease: Moderate Risk

- Male gender: Low Risk

Rationale: Multiple high-risk factors create cumulative risk for pressure injury development. Advanced age, diabetes, immobility, moisture from incontinence, and malnutrition significantly increase risk. Poor circulation from PVD and decreased kidney function add moderate risk. Gender alone doesn't significantly affect pressure injury risk (28).

Comprehensive Prevention Plan:

Positioning and mobility: Turn every 2 hours using 30-degree lateral position, avoid direct pressure on bony prominences, use pressure-relieving surfaces (foam mattress overlay), encourage chair sitting with position changes every hour.

Skin care: Keep skin clean and dry, use pH-balanced cleansers, apply moisturizer to dry areas (avoid over-moisturizing), inspect skin at least twice daily, manage incontinence promptly with barrier products.

Nutritional support: Consult dietitian for high-protein, high-calorie diet, encourage fluid intake (unless contraindicated), consider nutritional supplements, monitor albumin and prealbumin levels.

Environmental modifications: Use heel protectors or pillows to float heels, avoid shearing forces during position changes, use lift sheets for repositioning, maintain head of bed at lowest safe elevation.

Case Development: Mr. Peterson's care team implements an aggressive prevention protocol. The stage 1 pressure injury on his coccyx is treated with transparent film dressing and frequent position changes. Nursing staff ensures he's turned every 2 hours, even overnight, and uses proper technique to avoid shearing.

Dietary consultation leads to high-protein supplements and favorite foods from home to encourage intake. His incontinence is managed with scheduled toileting and barrier creams. Physical therapy begins gentle range-of-motion exercises and progressive mobility as his strength improves.

By discharge, his coccyx pressure injury has healed, and no new skin breakdown has occurred. His weight has stabilized, and he can transfer with minimal assistance.

Scenario 19: Basic Pain Management

Patient Background: Maria Santos, a 55-year-old office manager, presents to the pain management clinic for evaluation of chronic lower back pain that has been affecting her daily activities for eight months. The pain began gradually without specific injury and has progressively worsened despite conservative treatment with physical therapy and over-the-counter medications.

She describes her pain as a constant ache in her lower back with occasional sharp shooting pains down her left leg. The pain intensity varies from 4/10 in the morning to 7/10 by the end of her workday. Sitting at her desk for extended periods significantly worsens her discomfort, and she's had to modify her work station and take frequent breaks.

Ms. Santos has tried multiple approaches including physical therapy (6 weeks), chiropractic care, massage therapy, heat and ice applications, and various over-the-counter medications. She's concerned about taking prescription pain medications and prefers non-drug approaches when possible. The pain is affecting her sleep quality and her ability to participate in activities she enjoys (29).

Current Assessment: Ms. Santos appears comfortable at rest but grimaces when changing positions. Her vital signs are normal. Physical examination reveals muscle tension in the lumbar area, limited range of motion with forward flexion, and positive straight leg raise test on the left side. No neurological deficits are present in her lower extremities.

Pain Assessment Using Multiple Dimensions:

- **Intensity**: 6/10 current pain using numeric rating scale

- **Quality**: Aching, sometimes sharp and shooting

- **Location**: Lower back with radiation to left posterior thigh

- **Timing**: Constant with daily fluctuation, worse with prolonged sitting

- **Aggravating factors**: Sitting, bending forward, lifting

- **Relief factors**: Walking, lying down, heat application

- **Functional impact**: Difficulty with work tasks, sleep disruption, avoided activities

- **Emotional impact**: Frustration, worry about future progression

NGN-Style Highlighting Pain Descriptors:

Highlight the pain descriptors that suggest possible nerve involvement:

"Ms. Santos describes constant aching pain in her lower back that rates 4/10 in the morning and increases to 7/10 by evening. She experiences occasional sharp, shooting pains that travel down her left leg to her posterior thigh. The pain worsens with sitting and bending forward but improves with walking and lying down. She reports muscle stiffness and tension but no numbness or tingling in her legs."

Items to Highlight:

- sharp, shooting pains that travel down her left leg to her posterior thigh

- pain worsens with sitting and bending forward
- improves with walking and lying down

Rationale: Sharp, shooting pain with radiation down the leg suggests possible nerve root irritation or sciatica. The pattern of worsening with sitting and flexion, combined with improvement during walking, is consistent with lumbar disc involvement affecting nerve roots. This information guides further evaluation and treatment planning (30).

Comprehensive Pain Management Plan:

Non-pharmacological interventions: Continue physical therapy with focus on core strengthening, ergonomic workplace assessment and modifications, heat/cold therapy education, relaxation techniques for sleep improvement, gradual return to enjoyable activities.

Pharmacological options: Trial of NSAIDs with gastroprotection if no contraindications, muscle relaxant for acute exacerbations, topical preparations for localized relief, avoid opioids for chronic non-cancer pain without clear indication.

Lifestyle modifications: Weight management if appropriate, regular low-impact exercise program, sleep hygiene improvements, stress management techniques, pacing activities to prevent flare-ups.

Follow-up and monitoring: Pain diary to track patterns and triggers, functional assessment tools to measure improvement, regular reassessment of treatment effectiveness, consideration of additional interventions if conservative management fails.

Scenario 20: Medication Administration Safety

Patient Background: William Chen, a 68-year-old retired accountant, is hospitalized for management of acute heart failure exacerbation. He takes 12 different medications for multiple chronic conditions including heart failure, diabetes, hypertension, atrial fibrillation, and osteoarthritis. His medication regimen has become increasingly complex over the past two years as new conditions developed and treatments were added.

Mr. Chen admits to confusion about his medication schedule and acknowledges missing doses occasionally, especially when his routine is disrupted. His wife usually helps manage his medications at home, but she was hospitalized last month for hip replacement surgery. During that time, his medication adherence declined significantly, contributing to his current hospitalization.

His current medication list includes: furosemide 40 mg twice daily, lisinopril 20 mg daily, metoprolol 100 mg twice daily, warfarin 5 mg daily, metformin 1000 mg twice daily, insulin glargine 24 units at bedtime, aspirin 81 mg daily, atorvastatin 40 mg daily, omeprazole 20 mg daily, acetaminophen 650 mg as needed, and two over-the-counter supplements (31).

Current Assessment: Mr. Chen appears alert but somewhat overwhelmed when discussing his medications. His vital signs are stable following diuretic therapy. He can name most of his medications but is uncertain about dosing schedules and purposes for several drugs. He expresses anxiety about managing his complex regimen independently.

Medication Reconciliation Findings:

- **Home medications**: 12 prescription drugs plus 2 supplements

- **Potential interactions**: Warfarin with multiple drugs requiring monitoring

- **Duplicate therapy**: None identified

- **Inappropriate medications**: All appear appropriate for conditions

- **Administration complexity**: Multiple dosing schedules creating confusion

91

- **Patient knowledge gaps**: Limited understanding of drug purposes and side effects

High-Risk Medications Identified:

- **Warfarin**: Requires INR monitoring, multiple drug interactions, bleeding risk

- **Insulin**: Risk of hypoglycemia, especially with irregular eating

- **Furosemide**: Electrolyte imbalances, dehydration, fall risk from frequent urination

- **Metoprolol**: Bradycardia, hypotension, masking of hypoglycemia symptoms

NGN-Style Drag-and-Drop for Safety Checks:

Arrange the following medication safety checks in the correct sequence for administering Mr. Chen's morning medications:

Available Safety Steps:

- Check patient identification using two identifiers

- Verify medication orders against MAR (Medication Administration Record)

- Calculate dosages and check calculations with another nurse if needed

- Assess patient for contraindications (vital signs, lab values, symptoms)

- Explain medications to patient and verify understanding

- Document administration immediately after giving medications

- Observe patient for immediate adverse reactions

- Prepare medications using aseptic technique

Correct Sequence:

1. Check patient identification using two identifiers

2. Verify medication orders against MAR

3. Assess patient for contraindications (vital signs, lab values, symptoms)

4. Prepare medications using aseptic technique

5. Calculate dosages and check calculations with another nurse if needed

6. Explain medications to patient and verify understanding

7. Observe patient for immediate adverse reactions

8. Document administration immediately after giving medications

Rationale: This sequence follows the "Five Rights" of medication administration while incorporating safety checks at each step. Patient identification and order verification prevent wrong-patient errors. Assessment before preparation identifies contraindications. Proper preparation prevents contamination. Calculation verification prevents dosing errors. Patient education promotes adherence and safety awareness. Immediate documentation prevents double-dosing (32).

Comprehensive Medication Safety Plan:

Reconciliation and review: Complete medication history including over-the-counter drugs and supplements, identify potential interactions and duplications, assess appropriateness of each medication for current conditions, consider simplification opportunities.

Patient education: Review purpose of each medication, discuss common side effects and when to report concerns, demonstrate proper administration techniques, provide written information for reference.

Administration safety: Use two patient identifiers for every medication administration, verify orders and dosages before preparation, assess patient status before giving each medication, monitor for therapeutic effectiveness and adverse effects.

Discharge planning: Arrange medication synchronization to simplify pickup schedules, provide pillbox or medication management system, schedule follow-up appointments for monitoring, ensure understanding of when to contact healthcare providers.

Case Development: Mr. Chen's medication regimen is reviewed by the pharmacist and physician. Several medications are consolidated to twice-daily dosing when possible. His wife receives education about the medication management system before his discharge.

A pillbox system is provided with clear labeling for morning, noon, evening, and bedtime doses. Both Mr. and Mrs. Chen demonstrate understanding of the system and can identify high-risk medications requiring special monitoring. Follow-up appointments are scheduled for INR monitoring and medication effectiveness assessment.

Clinical Integration and Safety Culture

These safety scenarios demonstrate how fundamental nursing principles protect patients from preventable harm. Each situation requires systematic risk assessment, evidence-based interventions, and ongoing monitoring for effectiveness. The progression from individual patient safety (fall prevention) to system safety (medication administration) illustrates how safety thinking scales from bedside care to organizational processes.

Risk assessment skills: Students learn to use validated tools (Morse Fall Scale, Braden Scale) while understanding their limitations. Clinical judgment supplements standardized assessments by considering individual patient factors not captured in scoring systems.

Prevention strategies: Evidence-based interventions require adaptation to individual patient needs and preferences. Cookie-cutter approaches rarely work in complex patient situations requiring creative problem-solving within safety guidelines.

Interdisciplinary collaboration: Safety requires teamwork across disciplines. Physical therapy, pharmacy, dietary, and social services all contribute to comprehensive safety planning. Nurses coordinate these efforts while maintaining continuous bedside assessment.

Looking Ahead

Patient safety represents both a science and an art—it requires technical knowledge of risk factors and interventions combined with the wisdom to adapt these principles to individual patient situations. The scenarios in this chapter provide foundation skills that you'll build upon throughout your nursing career.

Remember that safety isn't about eliminating all risks—it's about making informed decisions that balance patient autonomy with protection from harm. Your role involves helping patients understand risks, providing education about prevention strategies, and creating environments that support safe care while maintaining dignity and quality of life.

The systematic thinking patterns you develop through these scenarios will serve you well as you encounter more complex safety challenges in advanced practice. Whether you're caring for critically ill patients in intensive care or managing community health programs, the fundamental principles remain the same: assess risks systematically, implement evidence-based interventions, monitor for effectiveness, and adjust your approach based on patient responses.

Key Learning Points

- Fall risk assessment uses validated tools but requires clinical judgment for individual patient factors

- Pressure injury prevention involves multiple interventions addressing risk factors and environmental modifications

- Pain management requires multidimensional assessment and individualized treatment approaches

- Medication safety follows systematic processes while adapting to complex patient regimens

- Risk factors often interact and compound, requiring comprehensive rather than single-intervention approaches

- Patient education plays crucial roles in all safety initiatives and requires assessment of individual learning needs

- Documentation provides communication tools for continuity of care and legal protection

- Evidence-based practice guides safety interventions but must be adapted to patient preferences and circumstances

- Interdisciplinary collaboration enhances safety outcomes through diverse expertise and perspectives

- Safety culture requires constant vigilance and commitment to continuous improvement in all care processes

Chapter 11: Complex Cardiovascular Scenarios

The sound of a code blue alarm pierces through the usual hospital noise, instantly transforming the peaceful medical unit into a coordinated response center. Intermediate-level cardiovascular scenarios test your ability to think quickly, prioritize effectively, and communicate clearly when minutes can mean the difference between life and death. These four complex situations—acute myocardial infarction, decompensated heart failure, new-onset atrial fibrillation, and hypertensive crisis—require you to integrate multiple assessment skills while coordinating care across healthcare teams.

Scenario 21: Acute Myocardial Infarction

Patient Background: Robert Martinez, a 58-year-old construction foreman, arrives at the emergency department via ambulance at 0800 after experiencing severe chest pain that started 45 minutes earlier while climbing scaffolding at a job site. He describes the pain as "crushing, like an elephant sitting on my chest" and rates it 9/10 in intensity. The pain radiates to his left arm and jaw, and he's been nauseated and diaphoretic since onset.

Mr. Martinez has a history of hypertension managed with lisinopril 20 mg daily and high cholesterol treated with atorvastatin 40 mg daily. He smoked one pack per day for 30 years but quit five years ago. His father died of a heart attack at age 62, and his brother had bypass surgery at age 55. He works physically demanding jobs and considers himself "in good shape" despite being 20 pounds overweight.

His coworkers report that he suddenly grabbed his chest, became pale, and started sweating profusely. He initially tried to "work through it" but agreed to call 911 when the pain didn't improve after 10 minutes. The paramedics administered aspirin 325 mg, established IV access, obtained a 12-lead EKG, and provided high-flow oxygen during transport (33).

Initial Assessment (0800): Mr. Martinez appears anxious and uncomfortable, clutching his chest. Vital signs show blood pressure 160/95, heart rate 105, respirations 24, temperature 98.6°F, and oxygen saturation 92% on room air. His skin is pale, cool, and diaphoretic. Heart sounds reveal regular rhythm with occasional premature beats. Lung sounds are clear bilaterally.

12-Lead EKG Findings: ST-elevation in leads II, III, and aVF (indicating inferior wall STEMI), with reciprocal changes in leads I and aVL. Q waves are beginning to form in leads III and aVF, suggesting acute inferior myocardial infarction with possible right ventricular involvement.

Laboratory Results (0820): Troponin I 0.8 ng/mL (elevated, normal <0.04), CK-MB 25 ng/mL (elevated), complete blood count normal, basic metabolic panel shows glucose 180 mg/dL, creatinine 1.0 mg/dL. Lipid panel pending.

NGN-Style Unfolding Case with Timed Decisions:

Time 0825 - Initial Interventions (Select all that apply): A. Administer nitroglycerin sublingual for chest pain B. Obtain IV access and begin normal saline at 125 mL/hr C. Apply oxygen at 4L nasal cannula D. Notify cardiology for emergent cardiac catheterization E. Administer morphine 2-4 mg IV for pain control F. Give clopidogrel 600 mg loading dose G. Start continuous cardiac monitoring

Correct Initial Interventions: B, C, D, F, G

Rationale: IV access is essential for medication administration and fluid resuscitation if needed. Oxygen supports tissue perfusion when saturation is below 94%. Cardiology notification enables rapid PCI (door-to-balloon time goal <90 minutes). Clopidogrel loading prevents further platelet aggregation. Continuous monitoring detects dangerous arrhythmias. Nitroglycerin is contraindicated in inferior MI due to possible right heart involvement and preload dependence. Morphine may be used cautiously but isn't first-line for STEMI (34).

Time 0835 - Condition Update: Mr. Martinez reports chest pain improved to 6/10 after interventions. Blood pressure has decreased to 140/85, heart rate 95. EKG shows continued ST elevation with new Q wave formation. Cardiology team is preparing for emergency cardiac catheterization.

Time 0835 - Next Priority Actions (Rank in order of priority):

1. Prepare patient for immediate cardiac catheterization

2. Continue cardiac monitoring and vital sign assessment

3. Administer additional medications per STEMI protocol

4. Notify family members of patient's condition

5. Complete admission assessment and documentation

Correct Priority Ranking: 1, 3, 2, 4, 5

Time 0845 - Pre-Catheterization: Patient reports chest pain now 4/10. Vital signs stable. Catheterization lab is ready. Patient expresses anxiety about the procedure and asks, "Am I going to die?"

Therapeutic Communication Response (Select best response): A. "Don't worry, everything will be fine. The doctors are very good." B. "I understand you're scared. The team is working quickly to open the blocked artery and restore blood flow to your heart." C. "You shouldn't think about that right now. Let's focus on getting you to the catheterization lab." D. "Many people have this procedure and do well. Try to stay positive."

Correct Response: B

Rationale: Acknowledges the patient's fear while providing factual information about the treatment goal. Avoids false reassurance while maintaining hope and explaining the purpose of the intervention (35).

Scenario 22: Decompensated Heart Failure

Patient Background: Margaret Chen, a 72-year-old retired librarian, presents to the emergency department with worsening shortness of breath, orthopnea, and bilateral lower extremity edema that has progressively worsened over the past week. She has a history of heart failure with reduced ejection fraction (HFrEF) following a myocardial infarction two years ago, managed with lisinopril, metoprolol, and furosemide.

Mrs. Chen reports sleeping in her recliner for the past four nights because she "can't breathe lying flat." She's gained 8 pounds in the past week despite following her prescribed low-sodium diet. Her daughter brought her to the hospital after finding her struggling to walk from the bedroom to the kitchen without stopping to rest.

Her current medications include lisinopril 20 mg daily, metoprolol succinate 100 mg daily, furosemide 40 mg daily, and spironolactone 25 mg daily. She admits to running out of furosemide three days ago and was unable to get to the pharmacy due to her increasing weakness. Her last echocardiogram six months ago showed an ejection fraction of 35% (36).

Current Assessment: Mrs. Chen appears anxious and in mild respiratory distress, using accessory muscles for breathing. Vital signs show blood pressure 95/65, heart rate 110, respirations 28, temperature 98.2°F, and oxygen saturation 88% on room air. Physical examination reveals jugular venous distension at 10 cm, bilateral crackles extending halfway up both lung fields, S3 gallop, and 3+ pitting edema to mid-calf bilaterally.

Diagnostic Results: Chest X-ray shows pulmonary edema with bilateral infiltrates and enlarged cardiac silhouette. BNP 2,400 pg/mL (severely elevated, normal <100). Basic metabolic panel reveals sodium 132 mEq/L, potassium 3.2 mEq/L, creatinine 1.4 mg/dL (baseline 1.0), BUN 45 mg/dL.

NGN-Style Matrix for Prioritizing Interventions:

Categorize the following interventions as "Immediate Priority," "High Priority," or "Moderate Priority":

Respiratory Support:

- Apply oxygen via nasal cannula to maintain saturation >92%: Immediate Priority

- Position patient in high Fowler's position: Immediate Priority

- Consider non-invasive positive pressure ventilation if no improvement: High Priority

Cardiovascular Management:

- Administer IV furosemide 80 mg (double home dose): Immediate Priority

- Monitor continuous cardiac rhythm: High Priority

- Assess response to diuretic therapy hourly: High Priority

Fluid and Electrolyte Management:

- Strict intake and output monitoring: High Priority

- Replace potassium to maintain level >4.0 mEq/L: High Priority

- Daily weights for fluid balance assessment: Moderate Priority

Patient Monitoring:

- Vital sign assessment every 15 minutes initially: Immediate Priority

- Assess lung sounds and work of breathing hourly: High Priority

- Monitor renal function during diuretic therapy: Moderate Priority

Rationale: Immediate priorities address life-threatening hypoxemia and acute pulmonary edema. High priorities support cardiovascular function and monitor treatment response. Moderate priorities provide ongoing assessment but aren't immediately life-threatening. The low blood pressure requires careful monitoring during diuretic therapy, as excessive diuresis can worsen hypotension and renal function (37).

Case Development: Mrs. Chen receives oxygen at 4L nasal cannula, improving her saturation to 94%. IV furosemide 80 mg produces 400 mL urine output in the first hour. Her respiratory status gradually improves, with decreased crackles and less accessory muscle use. Blood pressure remains stable at 100/70.

After four hours, she's produced 1,200 mL urine output, lost 3 pounds, and reports breathing "much better." Her potassium drops to 3.0 mEq/L, requiring replacement therapy. Creatinine increases slightly to 1.6 mg/dL, prompting adjustment of the diuretic dosing strategy.

Scenario 23: New-Onset Atrial Fibrillation

Patient Background: James Wilson, a 66-year-old retired engineer, presents to his primary care office for routine follow-up but reports feeling "fluttering" in his chest for the past three days. He describes episodes of rapid, irregular heartbeat that come and go, lasting 30 minutes to several hours. He's also noticed increased fatigue and mild shortness of breath with minimal exertion.

Mr. Wilson has a history of hypertension managed with amlodipine 10 mg daily and Type 2 diabetes controlled with metformin 1000 mg twice daily. He had a normal stress test and echocardiogram one year ago. He drinks 2-3 glasses of wine with dinner most evenings and has never smoked. His family history includes atrial fibrillation in his father at age 70.

He reports no chest pain, dizziness, or syncope. The palpitations don't seem related to physical activity or stress. He's concerned because his father had a stroke at age 75 that the family attributed to his heart rhythm problems. He's asking "Do I need to be on blood thinners like my dad was?" (38)

Current Assessment: Mr. Wilson appears comfortable but mildly anxious. Vital signs show blood pressure 145/88, heart rate irregularly irregular between 90-130 beats per minute, respirations 18, temperature 98.4°F, and oxygen saturation 96% on room air.

Cardiac examination reveals irregular rhythm with variable intensity S1, no murmurs. Lung sounds are clear. No peripheral edema noted.

12-Lead EKG Findings: Atrial fibrillation with rapid ventricular response, rate 115-135 bpm, no ST changes, QRS width normal. No signs of acute ischemia or ventricular hypertrophy.

Laboratory Results: Thyroid function tests normal (TSH 2.1 mU/L), basic metabolic panel normal, complete blood count normal, PT/INR normal at 1.0, HbA1c 6.8%.

NGN-Style Bowtie for Treatment Pathways:

Central Problem: 66-year-old male with new-onset atrial fibrillation with rapid ventricular response

Assessment Parameters (Select all appropriate):

- Calculate CHA2DS2-VASc score for stroke risk
- Assess hemodynamic stability
- Determine onset timeframe for anticoagulation decisions
- Evaluate for underlying triggers (hyperthyroidism, infection, alcohol)
- Monitor for signs of heart failure or ischemia

Rate Control Interventions (Select all appropriate):

- Metoprolol 25 mg twice daily
- Diltiazem 120 mg daily extended-release
- Digoxin 0.25 mg daily
- Cardioversion if hemodynamically unstable

Anticoagulation Decisions (Select all appropriate):

- Start warfarin with INR goal 2.0-3.0
- Consider direct oral anticoagulant (DOAC)

- Aspirin 81 mg daily for low-risk patients

- No anticoagulation if bleeding risk too high

Correct Selections: **Assessment**: All parameters appropriate for new-onset atrial fibrillation evaluation **Rate Control**: Metoprolol or diltiazem are first-line; digoxin reserved for specific situations; cardioversion not indicated for stable patient **Anticoagulation**: Calculate CHA2DS2-VASc score—this patient scores 3 points (hypertension, diabetes, age 65-74), indicating need for anticoagulation with warfarin or DOAC

CHA2DS2-VASc Score Calculation for Mr. Wilson:

- **C**ongestive heart failure: 0 points (no history)

- **H**ypertension: 1 point (on antihypertensive medication)

- **A**ge 65-74: 1 point

- **D**iabetes: 1 point (Type 2 diabetes)

- **S**troke/TIA history: 0 points (no history)

- **V**ascular disease: 0 points (normal stress test)

- **A**ge ≥75: 0 points

- **S**ex category (female): 0 points (male)

- **Total Score**: 3 points = High stroke risk, anticoagulation recommended

Treatment Plan: Mr. Wilson is started on metoprolol 25 mg twice daily for rate control and apixaban 5 mg twice daily for anticoagulation. His wine consumption is discussed as a potential trigger, and he agrees to limit alcohol intake. Follow-up is scheduled in one week to assess symptom improvement and medication tolerance (39).

Scenario 24: Hypertensive Crisis

Patient Background: Sandra Rodriguez, a 54-year-old high school principal, presents to the emergency department with severe headache, visual changes, and nausea that began 2 hours ago. Her blood pressure in triage is 220/118 mmHg. She has a 15-year history of hypertension but admits to poor medication adherence, often missing doses due to her busy work schedule and concerns about side effects.

Ms. Rodriguez stopped taking her antihypertensive medications (lisinopril and hydrochlorothiazide) three weeks ago because they made her "feel tired and dizzy." She's been under significant stress at work due to budget cuts and staff layoffs. She describes her current headache as "the worst I've ever had" and reports seeing "spots and flashing lights" in her vision.

Her medical history includes hypertension, hyperlipidemia, and a family history of stroke (mother at age 58) and heart disease (father at age 60). She's a non-smoker, drinks alcohol socially, and has gained 15 pounds over the past year due to stress eating and decreased physical activity (40).

Current Assessment: Ms. Rodriguez appears anxious and uncomfortable, holding her head. Vital signs show blood pressure 220/118, heart rate 95, respirations 22, temperature 98.8°F, and oxygen saturation 97% on room air. Neurological examination reveals mild confusion, bilateral papilledema on fundoscopic examination, and complaints of photophobia. Cardiac examination shows regular rhythm with S4 gallop. Lung sounds are clear.

Initial Diagnostic Results: Basic metabolic panel shows sodium 138 mEq/L, potassium 3.8 mEq/L, creatinine 1.8 mg/dL (elevated from baseline 1.0 mg/dL), BUN 35 mg/dL. Urinalysis shows 2+ protein, trace RBCs. Head CT scan shows no acute intracranial bleeding but mild cerebral edema.

Target Organ Damage Assessment:

- **Neurological**: Severe headache, visual changes, papilledema, mild confusion, cerebral edema on CT

- **Cardiovascular**: S4 gallop suggesting left ventricular hypertrophy

- **Renal**: Elevated creatinine, proteinuria, indicating acute kidney injury

- **Ophthalmologic**: Papilledema, visual disturbances

NGN-Style Trend Analysis with Interventions:

Blood Pressure Management Timeline:

Time 0900: BP 220/118 - **Intervention**: Establish IV access, begin continuous BP monitoring, neurological assessments every 15 minutes

Time 0920: BP 215/115 (no intervention yet) - **Intervention**: Start nicardipine infusion at 5 mg/hr, goal reduction 10-20% in first hour

Time 0940: BP 195/108 - **Assessment**: Appropriate reduction (11% decrease), continue current rate, monitor neurological status

Time 1000: BP 188/102 - **Assessment**: Continued improvement, neurological status stable, reduce nicardipine to 3 mg/hr

Time 1020: BP 175/95 - **Assessment**: Good response, headache improving, visual changes resolving

Target BP Goal: Reduce MAP by 10-20% in first hour, then gradual reduction to <180/110 over next 2-6 hours. Avoid precipitous drops that could cause cerebral or coronary ischemia.

Rationale: Hypertensive emergency requires careful BP reduction to prevent stroke, but overly aggressive treatment can cause watershed infarctions. The goal is controlled reduction while monitoring for improvement in end-organ damage symptoms. Nicardipine provides predictable, titratable BP reduction with rapid onset and offset (41).

Case Development: Ms. Rodriguez's blood pressure responds well to nicardipine infusion. Her headache improves significantly, visual changes resolve, and neurological examination returns to normal.

Renal function begins to improve with creatinine decreasing to 1.5 mg/dL by the next day.

She's transitioned to oral antihypertensive medications before discharge: lisinopril 20 mg daily and amlodipine 10 mg daily. Extensive patient education addresses medication adherence, lifestyle modifications, and the importance of regular follow-up. She's scheduled for outpatient appointments with cardiology and nephrology for ongoing management.

Clinical Reasoning Integration

These intermediate cardiovascular scenarios demonstrate the complexity of acute cardiac conditions requiring rapid assessment, prioritization, and intervention. Each case emphasizes different aspects of cardiovascular nursing: emergency response protocols, hemodynamic monitoring, medication management, and patient education.

The progression from STEMI (immediate life-threatening emergency) through heart failure exacerbation (complex fluid and medication management) to atrial fibrillation (chronic condition requiring anticoagulation decisions) and hypertensive crisis (careful titration of interventions) illustrates the range of clinical reasoning skills needed for cardiovascular nursing.

Key assessment skills: Recognition of cardiac emergencies, interpretation of diagnostic tests (EKGs, chest X-rays, laboratory values), hemodynamic assessment, and ongoing monitoring of treatment responses.

Intervention priorities: Time-sensitive treatments for STEMI, fluid management in heart failure, rate and rhythm control in atrial fibrillation, and controlled blood pressure reduction in hypertensive crisis.

Patient education needs: Understanding of chronic conditions, medication adherence importance, lifestyle modifications, and recognition of warning signs requiring immediate medical attention.

Professional Growth Opportunities

These scenarios prepare you for the rapid decision-making required in acute care settings. The ability to prioritize interventions, communicate effectively with healthcare teams, and provide patient education while managing complex medical conditions represents the essence of competent cardiovascular nursing practice.

Each case builds upon previous knowledge while introducing new concepts and decision-making challenges. The integration of assessment skills, clinical reasoning, and therapeutic interventions demonstrates how nursing expertise develops through exposure to increasingly complex patient situations.

The emphasis on patient education and long-term management reminds us that acute care episodes occur within the context of chronic disease management. Your role extends beyond immediate crisis intervention to include helping patients understand their conditions and make lifestyle changes that prevent future complications.

Looking Forward

Cardiovascular nursing requires a unique combination of technical skills, clinical judgment, and emotional support abilities. These scenarios provide foundation experiences that prepare you for more advanced practice situations while reinforcing the importance of systematic assessment, evidence-based intervention, and compassionate patient care.

The next section will challenge you with complex respiratory scenarios that require similar rapid assessment and intervention skills while introducing additional concepts related to oxygenation, ventilation, and respiratory failure management.

Key Learning Points

- STEMI requires immediate recognition and intervention with door-to-balloon time goals under 90 minutes

- Heart failure exacerbation management balances diuresis with maintaining adequate perfusion and renal function

- New-onset atrial fibrillation requires assessment of stroke risk using validated scoring systems and appropriate anticoagulation

- Hypertensive crisis demands careful blood pressure reduction to prevent end-organ damage while avoiding precipitous drops

- Multi-system assessment skills help identify complications and guide intervention priorities

- Continuous monitoring and reassessment allow for timely adjustments to treatment plans

- Patient education about chronic conditions and medication adherence prevents future acute episodes

- Time-sensitive interventions require efficient communication and coordination across healthcare teams

- Hemodynamic stability assessment guides the urgency and aggressiveness of interventions

- Evidence-based protocols provide frameworks while clinical judgment guides individualized care decisions

Chapter 12: Complex Respiratory Scenarios

Every breath represents a complex orchestration of muscle coordination, gas exchange, and cellular respiration that most people never consciously consider. But for patients experiencing respiratory compromise, each breath becomes a struggle that demands immediate nursing intervention and expert clinical judgment. These three challenging respiratory scenarios—COPD exacerbation with complications, pneumonia with sepsis risk, and post-operative respiratory complications—test your ability to assess oxygenation and ventilation while managing patients who may deteriorate rapidly without appropriate intervention.

Scenario 25: COPD Exacerbation with Complications

Patient Background: Harold Peterson, a 68-year-old retired mechanic, arrives at the emergency department via ambulance after his wife found him increasingly short of breath and confused at home. He has severe COPD (GOLD Stage 4) from a 45-year smoking history and has been hospitalized three times in the past year for exacerbations. His baseline functional status allows him to walk about 50 feet before needing to rest, and he uses home oxygen at 2 L/min continuously.

Mr. Peterson stopped smoking two years ago but continues to live in the same house where he smoked for decades. His current medications include tiotropium 18 mcg daily, salmeterol/fluticasone combination inhaler twice daily, albuterol as needed, and prednisone 10 mg daily for chronic inflammation. He completed a course of azithromycin one week ago for what his primary care provider thought was a respiratory infection.

His wife reports that he's been increasingly tired and confused over the past two days, with worsening shortness of breath that doesn't improve with his rescue inhaler. This morning, she found him sitting on the edge of the bed, unable to speak in complete sentences and appearing "blue around the lips." She's concerned because "he's never been this bad before" (42).

Initial Assessment: Mr. Peterson appears anxious and in severe respiratory distress, using accessory muscles and tripod positioning. Vital signs show blood pressure 155/95, heart rate 118, respirations 32 and shallow, temperature 100.2°F, and oxygen saturation 78% on his home oxygen at 2 L/min. His skin appears cyanotic, particularly around the lips and fingernails. He can only speak 2-3 words at a time before needing to breathe.

Physical Examination Findings: Barrel chest with increased anteroposterior diameter, diminished breath sounds bilaterally with expiratory wheeze throughout, prolonged expiratory phase, distant heart sounds, and use of accessory muscles including sternocleidomastoid and intercostal muscles. His mental status shows mild confusion with orientation to person and place but uncertainty about time.

Initial Diagnostic Results: Arterial blood gas on 2 L oxygen shows pH 7.28 (acidotic), PaCO2 68 mmHg (elevated), PaO2 52 mmHg (severely low), HCO3 28 mEq/L (compensated). Chest X-ray reveals hyperinflation with flattened diaphragms, increased retrosternal air space, and possible infiltrate in right lower lobe.

NGN-Style Unfolding Case with ABG Trends:

Time 1000 - Initial ABG Results:

- pH: 7.28 (Normal: 7.35-7.45)
- PaCO2: 68 mmHg (Normal: 35-45)
- PaO2: 52 mmHg (Normal: 80-100)
- HCO3: 28 mEq/L (Normal: 22-26)
- O2 Sat: 78%

Interpretation: Acute respiratory acidosis with partial metabolic compensation and severe hypoxemia

Immediate Interventions (Select all appropriate): A. Increase oxygen to 6 L nasal cannula to improve saturation B. Administer albuterol 2.5

mg via nebulizer
C. Give methylprednisolone 125 mg IV D. Prepare for possible BiPAP (bilevel positive airway pressure) E. Obtain sputum culture before antibiotics F. Start broad-spectrum antibiotic therapy

Correct Interventions: B, C, D, E, F (but NOT A)

Rationale: High-flow oxygen can worsen CO2 retention in COPD patients by reducing hypoxic drive and increasing V/Q mismatch. Bronchodilators and steroids address airway inflammation and bronchospasm. BiPAP can improve ventilation without intubation. Cultures guide antibiotic selection, but treatment shouldn't be delayed for culture results (43).

Time 1030 - After Initial Treatment: Mr. Peterson receives albuterol nebulizer, IV methylprednisolone, and is started on BiPAP at IPAP 12, EPAP 5. Oxygen is carefully titrated to maintain saturation 88-92%.

Repeat ABG Results:

- pH: 7.32 (improving)

- PaCO2: 62 mmHg (decreasing)

- PaO2: 68 mmHg (improving)

- HCO3: 28 mEq/L (unchanged)

- O2 Sat: 89%

Assessment of Response (Select best interpretation): A. Excellent response, continue current treatment B. Partial improvement, increase BiPAP settings C. Inadequate response, prepare for intubation D. Worsening acidosis, add bicarbonate

Correct Assessment: B

Rationale: pH and PaCO2 are improving but remain abnormal. Patient tolerance of BiPAP and gradual improvement suggest increasing settings may provide additional benefit before considering intubation. The goal is pH >7.30 and clinical improvement (44).

Time 1100 - Adjusted Treatment: BiPAP settings increased to IPAP 15, EPAP 6. Patient appears more comfortable, accessory muscle use decreased.

Follow-up ABG Results:

- pH: 7.35 (normalized)

- PaCO2: 58 mmHg (further improved)

- PaO2: 75 mmHg (adequate)

- HCO3: 29 mEq/L (stable)

- O2 Sat: 91%

This trend shows successful management of acute respiratory failure with non-invasive ventilation, avoiding the need for intubation while maintaining adequate oxygenation and improving ventilation.

Scenario 26: Pneumonia with Sepsis Risk

Patient Background: Dorothy Williams, a 75-year-old retired nurse, presents to the emergency department with a 4-day history of fever, productive cough, and increasing shortness of breath. She lives independently but has multiple comorbidities including diabetes mellitus (HbA1c 8.1%), chronic kidney disease stage 3, and heart failure with preserved ejection fraction. Her daughter brought her to the hospital because she seemed "more confused than usual" and had difficulty completing activities of daily living.

Mrs. Williams initially thought she had a cold and treated herself with over-the-counter medications. However, her symptoms progressively worsened, and she developed a productive cough with yellow-green sputum. Her daughter reports that her mother has been eating and drinking very little over the past two days and seems "not quite right mentally" (45).

Current Assessment: Mrs. Williams appears ill and slightly confused, oriented to person and place but unsure of the date. Vital signs show blood pressure 88/52 (baseline usually 130/80), heart rate 108, respirations 28, temperature 101.8°F, and oxygen saturation 90% on room air. Physical examination reveals decreased breath sounds and dullness to percussion over the right lower lobe with inspiratory crackles.

Laboratory Results: White blood cell count 18,500/μL with 85% neutrophils and increased bands, hemoglobin 10.2 g/dL, platelets 450,000/μL, glucose 245 mg/dL, creatinine 2.1 mg/dL (elevated from baseline 1.6), lactate 3.2 mmol/L (elevated), procalcitonin 8.5 ng/mL (markedly elevated).

Imaging Studies: Chest X-ray shows consolidation in right lower lobe consistent with pneumonia. No pleural effusion noted.

SIRS (Systemic Inflammatory Response Syndrome) Criteria Assessment:

1. **Temperature**: 101.8°F (>100.4°F or <96.8°F) ✓
2. **Heart rate**: 108 bpm (>90 bpm) ✓
3. **Respiratory rate**: 28 (>20 or PaCO2 <32) ✓
4. **White blood cell count**: 18,500 (>12,000 or <4,000 or >10% bands) ✓

Sepsis Assessment: Meets all four SIRS criteria plus suspected infection source (pneumonia) = **Sepsis diagnosis**

Severe Sepsis Indicators: Hypotension (systolic BP <90 or >40 mmHg below baseline), elevated lactate >2 mmol/L, altered mental status, acute kidney injury = **Severe sepsis**

NGN-Style Matrix for SIRS Criteria:

Evaluate the following assessment findings and categorize as "Meets SIRS Criteria," "Concerning but Not SIRS," or "Normal Finding":

Vital Sign Assessment:

- Temperature 101.8°F: Meets SIRS Criteria

- Heart rate 108 bpm: Meets SIRS Criteria

- Respiratory rate 28/min: Meets SIRS Criteria

- Blood pressure 88/52: Concerning but Not SIRS (indicates severe sepsis)

Laboratory Assessment:

- WBC 18,500 with increased bands: Meets SIRS Criteria

- Lactate 3.2 mmol/L: Concerning but Not SIRS (indicates tissue hypoperfusion)

- Glucose 245 mg/dL: Concerning but Not SIRS (stress hyperglycemia)

- Creatinine 2.1 mg/dL: Concerning but Not SIRS (acute kidney injury)

Clinical Assessment:

- Altered mental status: Concerning but Not SIRS (indicates organ dysfunction)

- Productive cough with purulent sputum: Normal Finding (expected with pneumonia)

- Decreased oral intake: Concerning but Not SIRS (contributing to dehydration)

Rationale: SIRS criteria include specific thresholds for temperature, heart rate, respiratory rate, and white blood cell count. Other findings indicate organ dysfunction (severe sepsis) or complications but don't meet SIRS definitions. Understanding these distinctions guides treatment intensity and monitoring requirements (46).

Sepsis Management Protocol:

Hour 1 (Golden Hour):

1. **Blood cultures** before antibiotics (but don't delay treatment >45 minutes)

2. **Broad-spectrum antibiotics** within 1 hour (ceftriaxone + azithromycin for community-acquired pneumonia)

3. **Fluid resuscitation** 30 mL/kg crystalloid for hypotension or lactate ≥4 mmol/L

4. **Lactate measurement** to assess tissue perfusion

5. **Oxygen therapy** to maintain saturation >92%

Ongoing Management:

- Vasopressors if hypotension persists after fluid resuscitation
- Source control (appropriate antibiotics for pneumonia)
- Supportive care for organ dysfunction
- Frequent reassessment for clinical response

Case Development: Mrs. Williams receives aggressive fluid resuscitation with 2 liters normal saline, broad-spectrum antibiotics, and oxygen therapy. Her blood pressure improves to 95/60, mental status clears somewhat, and oxygen saturation increases to 94%. Lactate decreases to 2.8 mmol/L after fluid resuscitation, indicating improved tissue perfusion.

Scenario 27: Post-Operative Respiratory Complications

Patient Background: William Johnson, a 62-year-old accountant, is 48 hours post-operative following elective open cholecystectomy (converted from laparoscopic due to adhesions). His surgery lasted 4 hours under general anesthesia, and his initial recovery was unremarkable. However, he's been reluctant to ambulate or perform deep breathing exercises due to incisional pain, despite adequate pain medication.

Mr. Johnson has a history of mild asthma (well-controlled with albuterol as needed), hypertension, and obesity (BMI 32). He's a former smoker (quit 10 years ago, 20-pack-year history) and works a sedentary job. His pain has been managed with morphine PCA and acetaminophen, but he's concerned about becoming "addicted" and has been using less pain medication than prescribed.

The nursing staff has noticed that his oxygen saturation has been trending downward over the past 12 hours, from 96% to 92% on room air. He complains of feeling "short of breath" and tired, and his incentive spirometry volumes have decreased from 2000 mL to 1200 mL. He's produced minimal sputum but reports feeling like he "can't take a deep breath" (47).

Current Assessment: Mr. Johnson appears comfortable at rest but becomes short of breath with minimal exertion. Vital signs show blood pressure 138/85, heart rate 92, respirations 24 and shallow, temperature 99.8°F, and oxygen saturation 89% on room air. Physical examination reveals diminished breath sounds at bilateral bases with fine crackles, especially on the right side.

Risk Factors for Post-Operative Pulmonary Complications:

- **Surgical factors**: Upper abdominal surgery, prolonged procedure (4 hours), general anesthesia

- **Patient factors**: Age >60, obesity, smoking history, inadequate pain control limiting mobility

- **Post-operative factors**: Reluctance to cough and deep breathe, limited mobility, shallow breathing pattern

Diagnostic Results: Chest X-ray shows bilateral lower lobe atelectasis with possible early infiltrate on the right. Arterial blood gas reveals pH 7.42, $PaCO_2$ 38 mmHg, PaO_2 68 mmHg on room air (A-a gradient widened). White blood cell count 11,800/μL (mildly elevated from baseline 7,500).

NGN-Style Highlighting Priority Actions:

Review Mr. Johnson's assessment data and highlight the findings that indicate need for immediate respiratory interventions:

"Mr. Johnson is 48 hours post-op from open cholecystectomy with oxygen saturation decreasing from 96% to 89% on room air over the past 12 hours. He reports shortness of breath and inability to take deep breaths. His incentive spirometry volumes have decreased from 2000 mL to 1200 mL. Physical examination reveals diminished breath sounds at bilateral bases with fine crackles, especially on the right side. He's been reluctant to ambulate or perform breathing exercises due to pain concerns. Temperature is 99.8°F and respiratory rate is 24 and shallow."

Priority Findings to Highlight:

- oxygen saturation decreasing from 96% to 89% on room air

- incentive spirometry volumes have decreased from 2000 mL to 1200 mL

- diminished breath sounds at bilateral bases with fine crackles, especially on the right side

- reluctant to ambulate or perform breathing exercises due to pain concerns

- respiratory rate is 24 and shallow

Rationale: These findings indicate developing atelectasis and possible pneumonia requiring immediate intervention. The combination of decreased oxygenation, reduced lung expansion, abnormal breath sounds, and shallow breathing pattern suggests significant respiratory compromise that will worsen without treatment (48).

Immediate Interventions:

Respiratory Support:

1. **Oxygen therapy** at 2-3 L nasal cannula to maintain saturation >92%

2. **Incentive spirometry** every hour while awake with coaching and encouragement

3. **Deep breathing and coughing exercises** every 2 hours with splinting support

4. **Chest physiotherapy** to mobilize secretions

Pain Management Optimization:

1. **Assess current pain level** and educate about importance of adequate analgesia for respiratory function

2. **Coordinate pain medication timing** with respiratory treatments and mobility

3. **Consider alternative pain strategies** (regional blocks, NSAIDs if appropriate)

4. **Reassure about appropriate pain medication use** for post-operative recovery

Mobility Enhancement:

1. **Progressive ambulation** starting with sitting on bedside, then walking in hallway

2. **Position changes** every 2 hours to promote drainage and ventilation

3. **Elevate head of bed** 30-45 degrees to optimize diaphragmatic excursion

Monitoring and Assessment:

1. **Oxygen saturation** continuous monitoring with alarms set

2. **Respiratory assessment** every 2-4 hours including breath sounds, work of breathing

3. **Temperature monitoring** for signs of infection development

4. **Chest X-ray** in 24 hours to assess progression

Case Development: Mr. Johnson's respiratory status improves with aggressive pulmonary hygiene measures and optimized pain management. His oxygen saturation increases to 94% on 2 L oxygen within 6 hours. Pain management consultation helps develop a multimodal approach that reduces his opioid requirements while maintaining comfort for respiratory exercises.

By post-operative day 4, his chest X-ray shows resolution of atelectasis, oxygen saturation returns to 96% on room air, and incentive spirometry volumes improve to 1800 mL. He's ambulating independently and demonstrates effective coughing and deep breathing techniques.

Clinical Integration and Respiratory Assessment Skills

These complex respiratory scenarios demonstrate the importance of systematic assessment, early recognition of deterioration, and prompt intervention to prevent respiratory failure. Each case emphasizes different aspects of respiratory nursing: acute exacerbation management, sepsis recognition and treatment, and post-operative complication prevention.

Advanced assessment skills: Interpretation of arterial blood gases, recognition of SIRS criteria, understanding of ventilation-perfusion relationships, and integration of subjective and objective findings to determine respiratory status.

Intervention priorities: Non-invasive ventilation for acute respiratory failure, sepsis bundle implementation for pneumonia with systemic involvement, and aggressive pulmonary hygiene for post-operative complications.

Patient education and advocacy: Understanding chronic disease progression, importance of medication adherence, recognition of early warning signs, and the role of pain management in post-operative recovery.

Evidence-Based Practice Applications

Each scenario incorporates current evidence-based guidelines: COPD exacerbation management using BiPAP and controlled oxygen therapy, sepsis bundle implementation within specified timeframes, and post-operative pulmonary complication prevention through multimodal interventions.

The progression from acute respiratory failure requiring advanced support through sepsis management requiring systematic protocol implementation to post-operative complication prevention through patient education demonstrates the range of clinical reasoning skills needed for respiratory nursing practice.

Moving Ahead

Respiratory nursing requires sophisticated assessment skills, understanding of pathophysiology, and the ability to intervene quickly when patients deteriorate. These scenarios prepare you for the complex decision-making required in acute care settings while emphasizing the importance of patient education and preventive interventions.

The next section will challenge you with multi-system scenarios that require integration of respiratory assessment skills with cardiovascular, neurological, and metabolic considerations— reflecting the reality that critically ill patients rarely have single-system problems.

Key Learning Points

- COPD exacerbations require careful oxygen management to avoid CO2 retention while treating acidosis and hypoxemia

- BiPAP provides effective non-invasive ventilation support for acute respiratory failure when properly titrated

- Sepsis recognition using SIRS criteria enables early intervention with antibiotics, fluids, and supportive care

- Post-operative pulmonary complications result from multiple factors requiring multimodal prevention strategies

- Arterial blood gas interpretation guides ventilation management and treatment effectiveness assessment

- Pain management significantly impacts respiratory function and recovery in post-operative patients

- Early mobility and aggressive pulmonary hygiene prevent many respiratory complications

- Continuous monitoring and reassessment allow for timely interventions and treatment modifications

- Patient education about chronic respiratory conditions improves long-term outcomes and prevents exacerbations

- Interdisciplinary collaboration enhances respiratory care through diverse expertise and coordinated interventions

Chapter 13: Managing Complex Medical Emergencies

The human body operates as an interconnected network where one system's failure creates cascading effects throughout the entire organism. These four multi-system scenarios challenge you to think beyond single-organ problems and consider how different body systems interact during critical illness. From diabetic ketoacidosis affecting metabolism, fluid balance, and neurological function to stroke with dysphagia threatening both neurological recovery and respiratory safety, these cases demand sophisticated clinical reasoning and coordinated care approaches.

Scenario 28: Diabetic Ketoacidosis

Patient Background: Jessica Martinez, a 28-year-old graduate student, arrives at the emergency department via ambulance after her roommate found her vomiting and confused in their apartment at 0600. Jessica has Type 1 diabetes diagnosed at age 16 and typically manages her condition well with insulin pump therapy. However, she's been under significant stress completing her master's thesis, working part-time, and dealing with her parents' recent divorce.

Her roommate reports that Jessica has been "acting strange" for the past two days—drinking excessive amounts of water, using the bathroom frequently, and complaining of stomach pain and nausea. Yesterday, Jessica mentioned that her insulin pump wasn't working properly, but she seemed too overwhelmed to deal with it immediately. This morning, the roommate found Jessica sitting on the bathroom floor, vomiting, and unable to answer simple questions coherently (49).

Initial Assessment: Jessica appears dehydrated and ill, with Kussmaul respirations (deep, rapid breathing) and a fruity odor to her breath. Her vital signs show blood pressure 95/55, heart rate 125, respirations 32 and deep, temperature 100.4°F, and oxygen saturation 98% on room air. She's oriented to person but confused about place and time, repeatedly asking "Where am I?" and appearing anxious and restless.

Physical Examination Findings: Poor skin turgor with tenting on chest and forearms, dry mucous membranes, sunken eyes, and delayed capillary refill of 4 seconds. Abdominal examination reveals diffuse tenderness without guarding or rebound. Her insulin pump shows "occlusion" error and appears to have been malfunctioning for approximately 18 hours based on pump memory.

Initial Laboratory Results:

- **Blood glucose**: 485 mg/dL (critically elevated)

- **Arterial blood gas**: pH 7.15 (severe acidosis), PaCO2 20 mmHg (compensatory hyperventilation), HCO3 8 mEq/L (severe metabolic acidosis)

- **Serum ketones**: 5.8 mmol/L (severe ketosis, normal <0.6)

- **Basic metabolic panel**: Sodium 128 mEq/L, potassium 5.2 mEq/L, chloride 95 mEq/L, BUN 35 mg/dL, creatinine 1.4 mg/dL

- **Complete blood count**: WBC 18,500/μL (stress response), hemoglobin 16.2 g/dL (hemoconcentration)

NGN-Style Unfolding Case with Lab Trends:

Time 0700 - Initial DKA Management:

Immediate Priorities (Rank in order):

1. Establish large bore IV access and begin fluid resuscitation

2. Start continuous insulin infusion protocol

3. Monitor cardiac rhythm for potassium changes

4. Begin hourly blood glucose and electrolyte monitoring

5. Assess mental status and neurological function

Correct Priority Ranking: 1, 2, 3, 4, 5

Rationale: Fluid resuscitation corrects severe dehydration and improves circulation. Insulin stops ketogenesis and reduces glucose. Cardiac monitoring detects dangerous potassium shifts. Frequent lab monitoring guides therapy adjustments. Neurological assessment monitors for cerebral edema (50).

Time 0800 - One Hour After Treatment Initiation:

Treatment Given:

- Normal saline 1 L over first hour

- Regular insulin 0.1 units/kg/hr continuous IV (7 units/hr for her 70 kg weight)

- Cardiac monitoring initiated

Follow-up Labs:

- **Blood glucose**: 420 mg/dL (decreased by 65 mg/dL)

- **pH**: 7.18 (slightly improved)

- **Serum ketones**: 5.2 mmol/L (beginning to decrease)

- **Potassium**: 4.8 mEq/L (decreasing as insulin works)

- **Sodium**: 130 mEq/L (corrected for hyperglycemia)

Next Priority Actions (Select all appropriate): A. Increase insulin infusion rate for faster glucose reduction B. Begin potassium replacement since level is trending down C. Continue current fluid rate with normal saline D. Add dextrose to IV fluid when glucose reaches 250 mg/dL E. Check blood glucose and electrolytes in one hour

Correct Actions: B, C, D, E (but NOT A)

Rationale: Glucose should decrease 50-75 mg/dL per hour—faster reduction risks cerebral edema. Potassium replacement prevents dangerous hypokalemia as insulin drives K+ into cells. Continued fluid replacement corrects dehydration. Dextrose prevents hypoglycemia while continuing insulin to clear ketones (51).

Time 1000 - Two Hours After Treatment:

Updated Labs:

- **Blood glucose**: 380 mg/dL (appropriate reduction rate)

- **pH**: 7.22 (continuing to improve)

- **Serum ketones**: 4.1 mmol/L (decreasing)

- **Potassium**: 4.0 mEq/L (requiring replacement)

- **Mental status**: More alert, oriented to person and place

Assessment Questions: Jessica asks, "What happened to me? Why do I feel so sick?" How should you respond?

A. "You had a serious diabetic emergency because your insulin pump wasn't working properly." B. "Don't worry about that now. Let's focus on getting you better." C. "Your blood sugar got very high and your body started breaking down fat for energy, which made you very sick." D. "You're in diabetic ketoacidosis. We're giving you insulin and fluids to fix the problem."

Best Response: C

Rationale: This explanation uses simple language to help Jessica understand what happened to her body without medical jargon, which supports her recovery and future prevention efforts while addressing her concern directly (52).

Time 1400 - Six Hours After Treatment:

Progressive Labs Show:

- **Blood glucose**: 180 mg/dL (now receiving D5 normal saline with insulin)

- **pH**: 7.35 (normalized)

- **Serum ketones**: 1.2 mmol/L (significantly improved)

- **Bicarbonate**: 18 mEq/L (improving)

- **Potassium**: 3.8 mEq/L (stable with replacement)

Transition Planning: Jessica's mental status has returned to baseline, she's tolerating oral fluids, and ketosis is resolving. The healthcare team discusses transitioning from IV insulin to subcutaneous insulin and addressing the factors that contributed to this episode.

Scenario 29: GI Bleed with Hemodynamic Changes

Patient Background: Robert Chen, a 65-year-old retired accountant, presents to the emergency department with a 2-day history of black, tarry stools and increasing weakness. He initially attributed his fatigue to "getting older" but became concerned this morning when he nearly fainted while standing up from bed. His wife noticed that he appeared pale and insisted on bringing him to the hospital despite his reluctance to "make a fuss."

Mr. Chen has a history of osteoarthritis managed with ibuprofen 800 mg three times daily for the past six months, hypertension controlled with lisinopril, and a remote history of peptic ulcer disease 15 years ago that was treated successfully. He denies abdominal pain, nausea, or vomiting, but reports feeling "dizzy and weak" especially when standing. He hasn't had any bright red blood in his stool or vomit (53).

Current Assessment: Mr. Chen appears pale and tired, lying quietly on the stretcher. His vital signs show blood pressure 85/55 (baseline usually 130/80), heart rate 110, respirations 20, temperature 98.2°F, and oxygen saturation 94% on room air. Orthostatic measurements reveal a blood pressure drop to 70/45 and heart rate increase to 135 when sitting up, with associated dizziness and diaphoresis.

Physical Examination: Pale conjunctiva and nail beds, delayed capillary refill of 3 seconds, cool extremities, and tachycardia with regular rhythm. Abdominal examination reveals mild epigastric tenderness without guarding or rebound. Digital rectal examination confirms melena (black, tarry stool) with no bright red blood.

Initial Laboratory Results:

- **Complete blood count**: Hemoglobin 7.2 g/dL (severely low, baseline 14.5), hematocrit 22% (severely low), platelets 380,000/μL

- **Basic metabolic panel**: BUN 55 mg/dL (elevated), creatinine 1.6 mg/dL (elevated from baseline 1.0), BUN/creatinine ratio 34 (suggests upper GI bleeding)

- **Coagulation studies**: PT 13.2 seconds (normal), INR 1.1 (normal)

- **Type and crossmatch**: Type A positive, crossmatched for 4 units packed red blood cells

NGN-Style Bowtie for Stabilization:

Central Problem: 65-year-old male with upper GI bleeding and hemodynamic instability

Assessment Parameters (Select all that apply):

- Serial hemoglobin and hematocrit levels

- Vital signs including orthostatic measurements

- Urine output monitoring

- Assess for signs of active bleeding

- Mental status and perfusion indicators

- Risk stratification using bleeding scores

Immediate Interventions (Select all that apply):

- Establish two large-bore IV lines (18 gauge or larger)

- Begin crystalloid fluid resuscitation

- Type and crossmatch for blood products

- Hold anticoagulants and NSAIDs

- Prepare for upper endoscopy

- Consider proton pump inhibitor therapy
- Insert Foley catheter for accurate urine output

Monitoring and Support (Select all that apply):

- Continuous cardiac monitoring
- Hourly vital signs and hemoglobin checks
- NPO status in preparation for endoscopy
- Fall precautions due to orthostatic hypotension
- Patient and family education about condition

Correct Selections: All listed items are appropriate for managing acute upper GI bleeding with hemodynamic compromise.

Hemodynamic Resuscitation Protocol:

Phase 1 - Initial Stabilization (0-30 minutes):

- Two 18-gauge IV lines established
- Normal saline bolus 500 mL over 15 minutes
- Blood type and crossmatch sent
- Gastroenterology consultation requested

Phase 2 - Ongoing Assessment (30-60 minutes):

- Hemoglobin rechecked: 6.8 g/dL (continuing to drop)
- Blood pressure improved to 95/60 after fluid resuscitation
- First unit of packed red blood cells started
- Upper endoscopy scheduled emergently

Phase 3 - Blood Product Administration: Mr. Chen receives 2 units of packed red blood cells over 4 hours with careful monitoring for transfusion reactions. His hemoglobin improves to 9.1 g/dL, blood pressure stabilizes at 110/70, and heart rate decreases to 88 bpm.

Endoscopy Findings: Upper endoscopy reveals a 1.5 cm duodenal ulcer with active bleeding (Forrest IIa classification), likely related to chronic NSAID use. The ulcer is successfully treated with injection therapy and thermal coagulation, achieving hemostasis.

Scenario 30: Acute Kidney Injury

Patient Background: Margaret Washington, a 70-year-old retired librarian, underwent contrast-enhanced CT angiography 48 hours ago to evaluate chest pain in the emergency department. The study ruled out pulmonary embolism, and she was discharged home with instructions for cardiology follow-up. However, she returns today with complaints of decreased urine output, mild nausea, and generalized weakness that has been worsening since yesterday.

Mrs. Washington has a medical history of diabetes mellitus type 2 (well-controlled with metformin), mild chronic kidney disease (baseline creatinine 1.4-1.6 mg/dL), and hypertension managed with lisinopril. She's been taking ibuprofen regularly for arthritis pain and admits to not drinking much fluid over the past few days because she "hasn't felt like it." She's concerned because she's only urinated twice since yesterday evening, and the amount was much less than usual (54).

Current Assessment: Mrs. Washington appears mildly dehydrated and tired. Her vital signs show blood pressure 155/92, heart rate 95, respirations 18, temperature 98.6°F, and oxygen saturation 96% on room air. Physical examination reveals mild peripheral edema in both ankles and decreased skin turgor. She reports feeling "foggy" and having difficulty concentrating.

Laboratory Results:

- **Current creatinine**: 3.2 mg/dL (baseline 1.4-1.6)

- **BUN**: 68 mg/dL (baseline 25-30)

- **Estimated GFR**: 18 mL/min/1.73m² (baseline 45-50)

- **Electrolytes**: Sodium 138 mEq/L, potassium 5.4 mEq/L (elevated), phosphorus 5.8 mg/dL (elevated)

- **Urinalysis**: Specific gravity 1.025, trace protein, few granular casts, no RBCs or WBCs

NGN-Style Trend Analysis of Renal Function:

Progression Timeline:

- **Baseline (3 months ago)**: Creatinine 1.5 mg/dL, BUN 28 mg/dL, GFR 48 mL/min

- **Pre-contrast study (48 hours ago)**: Creatinine 1.6 mg/dL, BUN 30 mg/dL

- **Current presentation**: Creatinine 3.2 mg/dL, BUN 68 mg/dL, GFR 18 mL/min

Analysis Questions: This pattern indicates: A. Chronic kidney disease progression (normal aging) B. Acute kidney injury superimposed on chronic kidney disease C. Laboratory error requiring repeat testing D. Dehydration causing falsely elevated values

Correct Answer: B

Rationale: The doubling of creatinine within 48 hours represents acute kidney injury (AKI) by definition. The timing following contrast exposure, combined with risk factors (diabetes, baseline kidney disease, NSAIDs, possible dehydration), suggests contrast-induced nephropathy superimposed on chronic kidney disease (55).

AKI Management Protocol:

Immediate Assessment:

1. **Fluid status evaluation**: Daily weights, intake/output monitoring, assessment for fluid overload

2. **Medication review**: Hold nephrotoxic drugs (NSAIDs, ACE inhibitors), adjust doses for kidney function

3. **Electrolyte monitoring**: Potassium, phosphorus, and acid-base status

4. **Urine output monitoring**: Goal >0.5 mL/kg/hr

Intervention Strategy:

- **Gentle fluid challenge** if dehydrated (250-500 mL normal saline)

- **Medication adjustments**: Hold metformin, lisinopril, and ibuprofen

- **Electrolyte management**: Kayexalate for elevated potassium if needed

- **Nephrology consultation** for further evaluation and management

Recovery Monitoring: Mrs. Washington's kidney function is monitored daily. Her creatinine peaks at 3.8 mg/dL on day 3, then gradually improves to 2.1 mg/dL by day 7. Urine output increases to normal levels, and she's discharged with nephrology follow-up and education about avoiding nephrotoxic medications.

Scenario 31: Stroke with Dysphagia

Patient Background: James Wilson, a 74-year-old retired engineer, was admitted 12 hours ago with acute ischemic stroke affecting the left middle cerebral artery territory. His wife found him at 0600 unable to speak clearly and with right-sided weakness. He received tissue plasminogen activator (tPA) within the therapeutic window and showed some neurological improvement, but significant deficits remain.

Mr. Wilson's medical history includes atrial fibrillation (poorly anticoagulated due to fall risk concerns), hypertension, and diabetes mellitus type 2. He was independent in all activities of daily living before this event and lived at home with his wife of 50 years. His current neurological deficits include right hemiparesis, expressive aphasia, and concerns about swallowing safety that have not yet been formally assessed (56).

Current Neurological Assessment:

- **Mental status**: Alert but frustrated, follows commands consistently

- **Speech**: Severe expressive aphasia, can say only a few words clearly

- **Motor function**: Right arm 2/5 strength, right leg 3/5 strength, left side normal

- **Sensation**: Decreased sensation on right side

- **Cranial nerves**: Right facial droop, possible swallowing difficulties

Swallowing Assessment Concerns: During medication administration, the nurse notices that Mr. Wilson coughs when drinking water and appears to have difficulty coordinating his swallow. Small amounts of water seem to remain in his mouth after swallowing attempts. His voice sounds slightly wet or gurgly after drinking, raising concerns about aspiration risk.

NGN-Style Matrix for Stroke Care Bundle:

Categorize the following interventions as "Immediate Priority," "High Priority," or "Moderate Priority" for Mr. Wilson's care:

Neurological Monitoring:

- NIH Stroke Scale assessment every 4 hours: High Priority

- Blood pressure monitoring and management: High Priority

- Neurological checks every 2 hours for first 24 hours: Immediate Priority

Swallowing and Nutrition:

133

- Keep NPO until swallow evaluation completed: Immediate Priority

- Speech-language pathology consult for swallow study: Immediate Priority

- Place IV line for hydration and medications: High Priority

- Consider nasogastric tube if prolonged NPO: Moderate Priority

Aspiration Prevention:

- Elevate head of bed to 30-45 degrees: Immediate Priority

- Suction equipment at bedside: High Priority

- Monitor for signs of aspiration pneumonia: High Priority

- Patient and family education about aspiration risks: Moderate Priority

Rehabilitation and Recovery:

- Physical therapy evaluation: High Priority

- Occupational therapy consultation: Moderate Priority

- Speech therapy for communication: Moderate Priority

- Discharge planning initiation: Moderate Priority

Rationale: Immediate priorities focus on preventing further neurological damage and aspiration. High priorities support recovery and monitor for complications. Moderate priorities address long-term recovery but aren't immediately life-threatening (57).

Comprehensive Stroke Care Plan:

Acute Phase Management (0-72 hours):

- Maintain NPO status until formal swallow evaluation

- Monitor neurological status for improvement or deterioration

- Blood pressure management per stroke guidelines

- DVT prophylaxis and skin integrity maintenance

- Early mobilization as tolerated

Swallow Assessment Protocol: Speech-language pathologist performs bedside swallow evaluation, noting impaired oral phase with delayed swallow initiation and possible silent aspiration. Modified barium swallow study confirms dysphagia with thin liquid aspiration risk.

Modified Diet Implementation:

- **Liquids**: Nectar-thick consistency to reduce aspiration risk

- **Solids**: Soft, minced texture with small bites

- **Positioning**: Upright at 90 degrees during and 30 minutes after meals

- **Supervision**: Nursing supervision during all oral intake initially

Case Development: Mr. Wilson's swallowing function gradually improves over 5 days with speech therapy interventions. He progresses from NPO to nectar-thick liquids and soft solids with supervision. His communication improves slightly, and he begins participating in physical and occupational therapy. He's discharged to acute rehabilitation with continued dysphagia precautions and ongoing speech therapy.

Clinical Integration and Multi-System Thinking

These multi-system scenarios demonstrate how complex medical conditions affect multiple organ systems simultaneously, requiring nurses to think broadly about patient care needs and coordinate interventions across different body systems. Each case illustrates how problems in one system create cascading effects throughout the body.

Systems Integration Skills: Understanding how diabetic ketoacidosis affects metabolism, fluid and electrolyte balance, cardiovascular function, and mental status. Recognizing how GI bleeding impacts circulation, perfusion, and multiple organ function. Appreciating how acute kidney injury influences fluid balance, electrolyte homeostasis, and medication metabolism.

Priority Setting Abilities: Managing competing needs when multiple systems require attention simultaneously. Determining which interventions must be implemented immediately versus those that can wait. Coordinating care across multiple specialties and healthcare team members.

Monitoring and Assessment: Recognizing early signs of complications that might affect multiple systems. Understanding how treatments for one problem might impact other organ systems. Maintaining vigilance for signs of clinical deterioration or improvement.

Professional Development Opportunities

These scenarios prepare you for the complexity of critical care nursing, where patients frequently have multi-system involvement requiring sophisticated clinical reasoning and coordination of care. The ability to think systematically about how different body systems interact during illness represents advanced nursing practice.

Each case builds upon previous knowledge while introducing new concepts about pathophysiology, pharmacology, and therapeutic interventions. The integration of assessment skills, clinical reasoning, and multi-system thinking demonstrates how nursing expertise develops through exposure to increasingly complex patient situations.

Broadening Understanding

Multi-system scenarios remind us that the human body functions as an integrated whole, not as isolated organ systems. Your role as a nurse involves understanding these connections and helping coordinate care that addresses all aspects of a patient's condition, not just the most obvious problems.

The emphasis on patient education, family involvement, and interdisciplinary collaboration reflects the reality that complex medical conditions require comprehensive approaches that extend beyond immediate medical treatment to include long-term management and prevention of complications.

These scenarios prepare you for advanced nursing practice where you'll encounter patients with multiple comorbidities, complex medication regimens, and treatment plans that must be carefully coordinated to avoid unintended consequences. The systematic thinking patterns you develop through these cases will serve you well throughout your nursing career.

Key Learning Points

- Multi-system conditions require understanding of how different organ systems interact during illness and recovery

- Diabetic ketoacidosis affects metabolism, fluid balance, cardiovascular function, and neurological status simultaneously

- GI bleeding management prioritizes hemodynamic stabilization while identifying and treating the source of bleeding

- Acute kidney injury requires medication adjustments, electrolyte monitoring, and nephrotoxic avoidance

- Stroke with dysphagia demands aspiration prevention while supporting neurological recovery and rehabilitation

- Priority setting becomes complex when multiple systems require immediate attention and interventions

- Laboratory trend analysis provides crucial information about treatment effectiveness and disease progression

- Patient education must address multiple aspects of complex conditions and their interactions

- Interdisciplinary collaboration ensures comprehensive care that addresses all aspects of multi-system conditions

- Recovery monitoring requires attention to multiple parameters across different organ systems

Chapter 14: Complex Medication Scenarios

Medications represent both our most powerful therapeutic tools and our greatest sources of patient harm—a paradox that defines modern healthcare practice. Each pill, injection, and infusion carries the potential to heal or hurt, and the difference often lies in the precision of dosing, timing, and monitoring that nurses provide. These four complex medication scenarios challenge you to think systematically about drug interactions, individual patient factors, and the delicate balance between therapeutic benefit and adverse effects.

Scenario 32: Anticoagulation Management

Patient Background: Harold Peterson, a 68-year-old retired machinist, was diagnosed with pulmonary embolism six weeks ago and started on warfarin therapy after initial treatment with enoxaparin. He presents to the anticoagulation clinic for routine INR monitoring and warfarin dose adjustment. His medical history includes atrial fibrillation, diabetes mellitus type 2, and osteoarthritis, which complicates his medication management due to multiple drug interactions and varying dietary habits.

Mr. Peterson's warfarin dosing has been challenging since initiation. His INR values have fluctuated between 1.8 and 3.6 over the past month, requiring frequent dose adjustments. He takes multiple medications that can influence warfarin metabolism, and his diet varies significantly based on seasonal vegetable availability from his home garden. Additionally, he's experienced minor bleeding episodes (increased bruising and occasional nosebleeds) that concern both him and his family (64).

Current Medication Regimen:

- Warfarin 5 mg daily (current dose, adjusted frequently)
- Metformin 1000 mg twice daily for diabetes
- Simvastatin 40 mg daily for hyperlipidemia

- Omeprazole 20 mg daily for GERD

- Acetaminophen 650 mg as needed for arthritis pain

- Multivitamin daily (contains vitamin K)

Recent INR History:

- Week 1: INR 2.1 (warfarin 5 mg daily)

- Week 2: INR 3.4 (warfarin reduced to 4 mg daily)

- Week 3: INR 1.9 (warfarin increased to 5.5 mg daily)

- Week 4: INR 3.1 (warfatin maintained at 5.5 mg daily)

- Today (Week 5): INR 2.8 (target range 2.0-3.0 for PE treatment)

Assessment of Factors Affecting INR Stability: Mr. Peterson reports that he's been more consistent with his diet lately, avoiding large amounts of leafy green vegetables after learning about vitamin K interactions. However, he admits to occasionally missing doses and sometimes taking extra doses if he "remembers" missing one. He's also started taking an herbal supplement (ginkgo biloba) that his neighbor recommended for memory, without informing his healthcare provider.

NGN-Style Cloze for Dosing Decisions:

Complete the anticoagulation management plan for Mr. Peterson:

"Based on Mr. Peterson's current INR of _____ and target range of _____ for pulmonary embolism treatment, his warfarin dose should be _____. The INR should be rechecked in _____ due to recent dose adjustments. His concurrent use of _____ may increase bleeding risk and should be _____. Patient education should focus on _____ and _____ to improve INR stability."

Answer Choices: 2.8, 2.0-3.0, maintained at current dose, 1 week, ginkgo biloba, discontinued, consistent dosing times, dietary consistency

Correct Completion: 2.8, 2.0-3.0, maintained at current dose, 1 week, ginkgo biloba, discontinued, consistent dosing times, dietary consistency

Rationale: INR of 2.8 falls within therapeutic range for PE treatment. Ginkgo biloba increases bleeding risk and should be discontinued. Consistent dosing and diet improve INR stability and reduce need for frequent adjustments (65).

Drug Interaction Assessment: Mr. Peterson's medications present several interaction considerations. Omeprazole can potentially increase warfarin effect by inhibiting CYP2C19 metabolism, though this interaction is generally mild. His multivitamin contains vitamin K, which could antagonize warfarin's effect, but the amount is typically small and effects can be managed with consistent daily intake. The newly added ginkgo biloba poses the most significant concern due to its antiplatelet effects, which could increase bleeding risk when combined with warfarin.

Patient Education Priorities:

Medication Adherence: Take warfarin at the same time each day, preferably in the evening. Use a pill organizer to track daily doses. Don't double up on missed doses—if you miss a dose and it's been more than 12 hours, skip it and resume normal schedule the next day.

Dietary Consistency: Maintain consistent vitamin K intake rather than avoiding it completely. You can eat leafy green vegetables, but try to eat similar amounts each week. Avoid cranberry juice and products, which can increase warfarin's effect significantly.

Bleeding Precautions: Use soft-bristled toothbrush, electric razor for shaving, and wear gloves during gardening. Watch for signs of serious bleeding including unusual bruising, prolonged bleeding from cuts, black tarry stools, or coughing up blood.

Drug Interactions: Always inform healthcare providers and pharmacists that you take warfarin before starting new medications, including over-the-counter drugs and herbal supplements. Some antibiotics, pain medications, and supplements can significantly affect your INR.

Scenario 33: Polypharmacy in Elderly

Patient Background: Eleanor Washington, an 80-year-old retired librarian, presents to the geriatric medicine clinic for medication review and management of her multiple chronic conditions. She currently takes 12 different prescription medications plus several over-the-counter supplements, and both she and her daughter are concerned about potential interactions and side effects. She's experienced several falls over the past three months, increased confusion, and frequent dizziness, particularly when standing.

Mrs. Washington lives independently in a senior apartment complex but relies on her daughter for transportation to medical appointments and pharmacy visits. She uses a weekly pill organizer but admits to occasionally forgetting doses or being unsure if she's already taken her medications. Her multiple physicians (cardiologist, endocrinologist, rheumatologist, and primary care) have each prescribed medications for their specific areas, but there's been limited coordination between providers (66).

Current Medication List:

1. **Metoprolol** 50 mg twice daily (hypertension, atrial fibrillation)

2. **Lisinopril** 20 mg daily (hypertension, heart failure)

3. **Furosemide** 40 mg daily (heart failure, edema)

4. **Warfarin** 3 mg daily (atrial fibrillation stroke prevention)

5. **Metformin** 1000 mg twice daily (diabetes mellitus)

6. **Glipizide** 10 mg twice daily (diabetes mellitus)

7. **Atorvastatin** 40 mg daily (hyperlipidemia)

8. **Omeprazole** 20 mg daily (GERD, gastroprotection)

9. **Tramadol** 50 mg three times daily (arthritis pain)

10. **Lorazepam** 0.5 mg at bedtime (anxiety, sleep)

11. **Diphenhydramine** 25 mg as needed for sleep

12. **Calcium carbonate** 500 mg twice daily (osteoporosis prevention)

Over-the-Counter Supplements:

- Multivitamin daily

- Vitamin D 1000 IU daily

- Fish oil 1000 mg daily

- Glucosamine/chondroitin for joint health

Recent Concerning Symptoms:

- Three falls in past three months (no serious injuries)

- Increased confusion and "foggy thinking"

- Dizziness when standing (orthostatic symptoms)

- Occasional nausea and decreased appetite

- Frequent urination, especially at night

- Dry mouth and constipation

NGN-Style Drag-and-Drop for Medication Reconciliation:

Categorize Mrs. Washington's medications based on their contribution to her current symptoms:

High Risk for Falls/Confusion:

- Lorazepam (sedating benzodiazepine)

- Diphenhydramine (anticholinergic effects)

- Tramadol (CNS depression, serotonin effects)

Contributing to Orthostatic Hypotension:

- Metoprolol (beta-blocker effects)
- Lisinopril (ACE inhibitor effects)
- Furosemide (volume depletion)

Potential Drug Interactions:

- Warfarin + multiple medications (bleeding risk)
- Tramadol + other CNS depressants
- Calcium + other medications (absorption interference)

Anticholinergic Burden (dry mouth, constipation, confusion):

- Diphenhydramine (high anticholinergic activity)
- Tramadol (moderate anticholinergic effects)

Medication Optimization Plan:

Immediate Discontinuations:

1. **Diphenhydramine**: High anticholinergic burden contributing to confusion and falls. Replace with sleep hygiene education and melatonin if needed.
2. **Lorazepam**: Benzodiazepine increases fall risk in elderly. Taper slowly and consider non-pharmacological anxiety management.

Dose Reductions:

1. **Tramadol**: Reduce to twice daily or consider topical NSAIDs for arthritis pain to decrease CNS effects.
2. **Furosemide**: Assess if current dose necessary; may contribute to orthostatic hypotension.

Medication Timing Optimization:

1. **Metoprolol and Lisinopril**: Consider taking at bedtime to reduce daytime orthostatic effects.

2. **Calcium carbonate**: Separate from other medications by 2 hours to prevent absorption interactions.

Alternative Considerations:

1. **Sleep management**: Sleep hygiene education, evening routine, possible melatonin trial instead of sedating medications.

2. **Pain management**: Physical therapy referral, topical treatments, acetaminophen around-the-clock for arthritis.

Scenario 34: Insulin Management Challenges

Patient Background: Maria Santos, a 55-year-old office manager, has had Type 1 diabetes for 28 years and typically maintains good glycemic control with insulin pump therapy. However, over the past three months, her blood glucose readings have become increasingly erratic, ranging from severe hypoglycemia (requiring glucagon administration twice) to persistent hyperglycemia despite aggressive insulin adjustments. Her most recent HbA1c increased from 7.2% to 8.8%, indicating significant deterioration in control.

Ms. Santos attributes her glucose variability to increased work stress (recent promotion to management position), irregular eating patterns due to long meetings, and disrupted sleep schedules. She's also been dealing with her teenage daughter's behavioral problems and her elderly mother's increasing care needs. Additionally, she's gained 12 pounds over the past year and wonders if this affects her insulin sensitivity (67).

Current Insulin Regimen (via insulin pump):

- **Basal rates**: 0.8 units/hour from midnight to 6 AM, 1.2 units/hour from 6 AM to 10 PM

- **Carbohydrate ratio**: 1 unit per 12 grams carbohydrate

- **Correction factor**: 1 unit per 40 mg/dL above 120 mg/dL target

- **Total daily insulin**: Averaging 45-55 units (increased from previous 38-42 units)

Recent Blood Glucose Patterns (2-week period):

- **Fasting glucose**: Range 85-245 mg/dL, average 165 mg/dL

- **Pre-meal readings**: Highly variable, 70-320 mg/dL

- **Post-meal peaks**: Often exceeding 300 mg/dL, even with pre-bolus timing

- **Overnight lows**: Three episodes below 60 mg/dL, including two severe episodes requiring treatment

- **Dawn phenomenon**: Significant morning rise from 3 AM to 7 AM

Lifestyle Factor Analysis: Ms. Santos works 50-60 hours per week in a demanding management role. Her eating schedule varies dramatically—sometimes skipping breakfast, eating lunch at her desk while working, and having dinner as late as 9 PM. She exercises sporadically (previously ran 3-4 times weekly, now maybe once per week). Her sleep quality is poor, averaging 5-6 hours nightly with frequent awakenings due to work stress and family concerns.

NGN-Style Trend Analysis with Insulin Adjustments:

Week 1 Glucose Pattern Analysis:

- **Monday**: Fasting 145, lunch 280 (despite calculated bolus), dinner 95, bedtime 180

- **Tuesday**: Fasting 200, skipped lunch, dinner 320, bedtime 150

- **Wednesday**: Fasting 85, lunch 250, dinner 75 (severe low), bedtime 160

- **Thursday**: Fasting 165, lunch 195, dinner 240, bedtime 185

- **Friday**: Fasting 220, lunch 300, dinner 160, bedtime 175

Insulin Adjustment Strategy:

Basal Rate Modifications:

- Increase overnight basal from 0.8 to 1.0 units/hour to address dawn phenomenon
- Consider temporary basal rate increases during high-stress work periods
- Add additional basal rate from 3 AM to 8 AM at 1.4 units/hour for dawn phenomenon

Bolus Ratio Adjustments:

- Adjust carbohydrate ratio from 1:12 to 1:10 for breakfast and lunch (increased insulin resistance)
- Modify correction factor from 1:40 to 1:35 for more aggressive correction
- Implement extended bolus for high-fat meals that cause delayed glucose spikes

Timing and Technique Improvements:

- Pre-bolus 15-20 minutes before meals when glucose is elevated
- Use temporary basal rate reductions for delayed or skipped meals
- Set pump alarms for missed bolus reminders during busy work periods

Lifestyle Integration Strategies:

Meal Planning and Timing:

1. Prepare consistent breakfast options that can be eaten quickly

2. Schedule protected lunch time with consistent carbohydrate content

3. Plan dinner timing to avoid late-night eating when possible

4. Keep glucose tablets and protein snacks readily available

Stress Management Impact:

1. **Exercise resumption**: Start with 20-minute walks during lunch breaks, gradually increase to previous running routine

2. **Sleep hygiene**: Establish consistent bedtime routine, limit work-related activities 2 hours before bed

3. **Stress reduction**: Consider counseling or stress management classes to address work and family pressures

Technology Utilization:

1. Use continuous glucose monitor integration with pump for better trend awareness

2. Set customized alarms for glucose thresholds based on activity and meal timing

3. Use smartphone apps for carbohydrate counting accuracy during busy periods

Scenario 35: Pain Crisis Management

Patient Background: Robert Johnson, a 45-year-old construction supervisor, presents to the emergency department in sickle cell pain crisis—his fourth hospitalization this year. He has sickle cell disease (HbSS) diagnosed in childhood and typically experiences 6-8 pain crises annually, usually triggered by dehydration, infection, or physical stress. His current crisis began 18 hours ago with severe pain in his back, chest, and both legs, rating his pain as 9/10 despite taking his home pain medications.

Mr. Johnson works in construction despite his condition, which often leads to dehydration and physical stress that trigger crises. He's developed tolerance to opioid pain medications over his 30+ years of managing sickle cell disease, requiring increasingly higher doses for adequate pain relief. He's also frustrated with emergency department staff who sometimes question the legitimacy of his pain or are reluctant to provide adequate pain medication due to concerns about drug-seeking behavior (68).

Current Pain Assessment:

- **Pain intensity**: 9/10 on numeric rating scale

- **Pain quality**: Deep, aching, throbbing in bones and joints

- **Pain location**: Lower back, chest, bilateral legs (typical crisis pattern)

- **Pain triggers**: Recent dehydration from hot weather work conditions

- **Functional impact**: Unable to walk without assistance, cannot lie comfortably

- **Previous effective treatments**: IV morphine, hydromorphone, aggressive hydration

Home Medication Regimen:

- **Hydrocodone/acetaminophen** 10/325 mg every 4-6 hours for pain

- **Ibuprofen** 800 mg three times daily for inflammation

- **Folic acid** 1 mg daily for red blood cell production

- **Hydroxurea** 500 mg daily (disease-modifying therapy)

Current Vital Signs and Assessment:

- Blood pressure 155/95 (elevated due to pain)

- Heart rate 110 (elevated due to pain and possible dehydration)

- Respirations 22 (slightly elevated)

- Temperature 99.2°F (low-grade fever common in crisis)

- Oxygen saturation 94% on room air (concerning, may indicate acute chest syndrome)

Laboratory Results:

- Hemoglobin 7.8 g/dL (baseline 8-9 g/dL for this patient)

- White blood cell count 15,500/µL (elevated, indicating stress response)

- Reticulocyte count 8% (elevated, indicating increased red cell production)

- Lactate dehydrogenase 450 U/L (elevated, indicating hemolysis)

- Bilirubin 3.2 mg/dL (elevated, indicating increased red cell breakdown)

NGN-Style Highlighting Pain Interventions:

Review Mr. Johnson's pain crisis presentation and highlight the interventions that should be prioritized:

"Mr. Johnson presents with severe sickle cell pain crisis rating 9/10, located in back, chest, and legs. His vital signs show blood pressure 155/95, heart rate 110, and oxygen saturation 94% on room air. He has a history of multiple hospitalizations and requires high-dose opioids for adequate pain relief. His home medications include hydrocodone/acetaminophen and ibuprofen. Laboratory results show hemoglobin 7.8 g/dL and elevated markers of hemolysis. He appears dehydrated and reports the crisis began after working in hot weather conditions."

Priority Interventions to Highlight:

- IV access and aggressive fluid resuscitation for dehydration

- High-dose opioid analgesia (morphine or hydromorphone IV)

- Oxygen therapy to maintain saturation above 95%

- Monitor for acute chest syndrome development

- Avoid medications that may precipitate sickling (meperidine)

Rationale: Sickle cell crisis requires aggressive pain management with opioids, as patients develop tolerance and require higher doses. Fluid resuscitation prevents further sickling. Oxygen saturation of 94% is concerning for possible acute chest syndrome. Early aggressive treatment prevents complications (69).

Multimodal Pain Management Protocol:

Pharmacological Interventions:

Primary Analgesics:

1. **Morphine 0.1-0.15 mg/kg IV** every 2-4 hours (approximately 8-12 mg for 70 kg patient)

2. **Hydromorphone 1-2 mg IV** every 2-4 hours as alternative to morphine

3. **Patient-controlled analgesia (PCA)** pump for consistent dosing

Adjuvant Medications:

1. **Ketorolac 30 mg IV** every 6 hours for anti-inflammatory effect (limit to 5 days)

2. **Acetaminophen 1000 mg** every 6 hours for additional analgesia

3. **Gabapentin or pregabalin** for neuropathic pain component

Supportive Care:

1. **Normal saline infusion** at 1.5 times maintenance rate for rehydration

2. **Oxygen therapy** to maintain saturation above 95%

3. **Heat application** to affected areas for comfort

Non-Pharmacological Interventions:

Comfort Measures:

1. **Positioning**: Support painful areas with pillows, encourage position changes

2. **Environmental modifications**: Quiet room, dim lighting, temperature control

3. **Distraction techniques**: Music, television, reading materials as tolerated

Psychosocial Support:

1. **Pain validation**: Acknowledge legitimacy of pain, avoid judgmental attitudes

2. **Anxiety management**: Reassurance, relaxation techniques, possibly anxiolytics

3. **Family involvement**: Include family members in care planning and education

Monitoring and Assessment:

Pain Response Monitoring:

- Reassess pain intensity every 2 hours initially, then every 4 hours

- Document pain character, location, and functional impact

- Monitor for breakthrough pain requiring additional medication

- Assess effectiveness of interventions and adjust as needed

Complication Monitoring:

- Watch for signs of acute chest syndrome (chest pain, dyspnea, new infiltrates on X-ray)

- Monitor for signs of infection that could worsen crisis

- Assess hydration status and urine output

- Watch for signs of stroke or other neurological complications

Case Development: Mr. Johnson receives aggressive pain management with IV morphine PCA, achieving pain reduction to 4-5/10 within 6 hours. His oxygen saturation improves to 96% with supplemental oxygen, and no signs of acute chest syndrome develop. He's discharged after 48 hours with improved pain control and education about crisis prevention strategies.

Medication Safety and Clinical Expertise

These complex medication scenarios demonstrate the sophisticated knowledge and clinical reasoning required for safe medication management in challenging patient situations. Each case illustrates how individual patient factors, drug interactions, and clinical circumstances influence medication decisions and monitoring requirements.

Advanced Pharmacology Application: Understanding how patient age, comorbidities, and concurrent medications affect drug metabolism, distribution, and elimination. Recognizing when standard dosing guidelines need modification based on individual patient factors.

Risk Assessment and Mitigation: Identifying patients at high risk for adverse drug events and implementing monitoring strategies to detect problems early. Balancing therapeutic benefits with potential harm in complex medication regimens.

Patient Education and Advocacy: Helping patients understand their medications, recognize adverse effects, and participate actively in their medication management. Advocating for appropriate pain management and addressing barriers to adherence.

Professional Development Through Medication Expertise

These scenarios prepare you for advanced nursing practice where medication management represents a significant portion of your clinical responsibilities. The ability to assess drug interactions, monitor for adverse effects, and optimize therapeutic regimens requires both scientific knowledge and clinical judgment.

Each case builds upon fundamental pharmacology principles while introducing real-world complexities that textbooks rarely address. The integration of medication knowledge with assessment skills, patient education, and interdisciplinary collaboration demonstrates the breadth of expertise required for competent medication management.

Reflections on Therapeutic Relationships

Medication management extends far beyond simply administering drugs according to prescribed protocols. These scenarios illustrate how therapeutic relationships, patient education, and individualized care planning contribute to successful medication outcomes. Your role includes not just ensuring safe administration, but helping patients understand their therapies, manage side effects, and achieve optimal therapeutic benefits.

The emphasis on patient advocacy, particularly evident in the sickle cell pain management scenario, reminds us that nurses serve as crucial bridges between patients and healthcare systems, ensuring that individual needs are met within the context of evidence-based practice guidelines.

These complex medication scenarios prepare you for the realities of modern healthcare, where patients frequently take multiple medications, have complex medical histories, and require individualized approaches to achieve optimal therapeutic outcomes while minimizing harm.

Key Learning Points

- Anticoagulation management requires understanding of drug interactions, dietary factors, and patient-specific variables affecting INR stability

- Polypharmacy in elderly patients demands systematic medication review and deprescribing to reduce adverse effects and drug interactions

- Insulin management challenges require integration of blood glucose patterns with lifestyle factors and stress management strategies

- Sickle cell pain crisis management requires aggressive multimodal analgesia and understanding of disease-specific pain characteristics

- Medication reconciliation involves more than listing drugs—it requires analysis of therapeutic appropriateness and potential interactions

- Patient education plays a crucial role in medication adherence and safety monitoring

- Individual patient factors significantly influence medication dosing, monitoring, and expected responses

- Technology integration (pumps, monitors, apps) enhances medication management but requires clinical expertise for optimal utilization

- Interdisciplinary collaboration ensures comprehensive medication management across multiple providers and care settings

- Advocacy for appropriate medication management includes addressing provider biases and patient access barriers

Chapter 15: Advanced Critical Care Scenarios

The shrill sound of multiple alarms creates a symphony of urgency that transforms the intensive care unit into a coordinated battlefield against critical illness. Advanced-level scenarios test not only your clinical knowledge but your leadership abilities, ethical reasoning, and capacity to make life-and-death decisions under extreme pressure. These situations—from cardiogenic shock requiring mechanical support to code blue leadership during cardiac arrest—demand the highest levels of nursing expertise and professional judgment.

Scenario 36: Cardiogenic Shock

Patient Background: Michael Rodriguez, a 62-year-old construction supervisor, arrives in the coronary care unit following emergency cardiac catheterization for a massive anterior wall STEMI. Despite successful primary percutaneous coronary intervention (PCI) to his completely occluded left anterior descending artery, he continues to show signs of severe left ventricular dysfunction and cardiogenic shock. His ejection fraction on bedside echocardiogram is estimated at 20%, and he requires multiple vasoactive medications to maintain adequate blood pressure.

Mr. Rodriguez's medical history includes mild hypertension and hyperlipidemia, but he was otherwise healthy and working full-time until this event. He has no prior history of heart disease, though his father died of a heart attack at age 58. The catheterization revealed that the large LAD supplied a significant portion of his left ventricle, and despite successful reperfusion, the damage appears extensive (58).

Current Assessment: Mr. Rodriguez is intubated and sedated, requiring mechanical ventilation due to pulmonary edema and respiratory failure. His hemodynamic parameters show profound cardiovascular compromise with systolic blood pressure maintained at 85-90 mmHg only with high-dose vasoactive support. A pulmonary artery catheter has been inserted for precise hemodynamic monitoring.

Hemodynamic Profile:

- **Blood pressure**: 88/55 mmHg (on multiple pressors)

- **Heart rate**: 110 bpm with occasional premature ventricular contractions

- **Central venous pressure**: 18 mmHg (elevated, indicating right heart failure)

- **Pulmonary capillary wedge pressure**: 28 mmHg (severely elevated, indicating left heart failure)

- **Cardiac output**: 3.2 L/min (severely reduced, normal 4-8 L/min)

- **Cardiac index**: 1.6 L/min/m² (severely reduced, normal 2.5-4.0)

- **Systemic vascular resistance**: 2800 dynes·sec·cm^{-5} (elevated due to vasoconstriction)

Current Medications: Norepinephrine 0.15 mcg/kg/min, dobutamine 7.5 mcg/kg/min, milrinone 0.4 mcg/kg/min, furosemide drip 5 mg/hr, and heparin per protocol.

NGN-Style Complex Unfolding Case:

Hour 1 - Initial ICU Management:

Priority Assessment Parameters (Select all appropriate): A. Continuous arterial blood pressure monitoring B. Hourly urine output measurement C. Serial lactate levels to assess tissue perfusion D. Echocardiogram to assess ventricular function E. Chest X-ray to evaluate pulmonary edema F. Mixed venous oxygen saturation monitoring

Correct Selections: All listed parameters are appropriate for cardiogenic shock management.

Hour 3 - Worsening Clinical Status: Despite maximum medical therapy, Mr. Rodriguez shows signs of deterioration. His cardiac output has decreased to 2.8 L/min, lactate has increased from 3.2 to 4.8 mmol/L, and urine output has dropped to 15 mL/hr for the past two hours. The cardiothoracic surgery team has been consulted for possible mechanical circulatory support.

Next Level Interventions (Rank in order of urgency):

1. Prepare for intra-aortic balloon pump (IABP) insertion

2. Consider escalation to Impella or ECMO support

3. Optimize current vasoactive medication regimens

4. Increase diuretic therapy for fluid management

5. Evaluate for additional coronary lesions

Correct Ranking: 1, 3, 2, 5, 4

Rationale: IABP provides immediate hemodynamic support by reducing afterload and improving coronary perfusion. Medication optimization should occur simultaneously. Advanced mechanical support (Impella/ECMO) may be needed if IABP insufficient. Evaluation for additional lesions guides further intervention. Diuresis is lowest priority in shock state (59).

Hour 6 - Post-IABP Insertion: An intra-aortic balloon pump has been successfully inserted via the right femoral artery. The device is functioning appropriately with 1:1 assist ratio, and hemodynamic parameters show modest improvement.

Updated Hemodynamics:

- **Blood pressure**: 95/60 mmHg (improved)

- **Cardiac output**: 3.8 L/min (improved)

- **Lactate**: 4.2 mmol/L (beginning to improve)

- **Urine output**: 25 mL/hr (improved)

IABP Management Priorities:

- Monitor balloon pump timing and function continuously

- Assess circulation to affected extremity every hour

- Maintain strict bed rest with affected leg straight

- Prevent thrombosis with anticoagulation per protocol

- Watch for balloon pump complications (bleeding, limb ischemia, hemolysis)

Case Development: Mr. Rodriguez's condition stabilizes over the next 48 hours with IABP support. His cardiac output improves to 4.2 L/min, lactate normalizes, and kidney function begins to recover. The IABP is gradually weaned over 72 hours as his native cardiac function shows signs of recovery, though he will require long-term heart failure management.

Scenario 37: Multi-Vessel Cardiac Disease

Patient Background: Robert Chen, a 68-year-old retired engineer, presents to the emergency department with chest pain that began during his morning walk and has persisted for 90 minutes despite rest and sublingual nitroglycerin. Unlike his previous episodes of stable angina, this pain feels "different"—more intense, radiating to both arms, and accompanied by nausea and diaphoresis. His wife insisted on calling 911 when she found him sitting pale and sweaty on their front steps, unable to catch his breath.

Mr. Chen has a 12-year history of coronary artery disease with previous percutaneous coronary intervention to his right coronary artery five years ago. His current medications include dual antiplatelet therapy (aspirin and clopidogrel), atorvastatin, metoprolol, and lisinopril. Despite good medication adherence and lifestyle modifications, his cardiologist has been monitoring progressive disease in his left anterior descending and circumflex arteries, with plans for elective intervention "when symptoms warrant it" (75).

Current Assessment: Mr. Chen appears anxious and uncomfortable, with obvious signs of sympathetic activation. His vital signs show blood pressure 165/95 (elevated from his usual 130/80), heart rate 105, respirations 22, temperature 98.4°F, and oxygen saturation 94% on room air. Physical examination reveals diaphoresis, cool extremities, and an S4 gallop suggestive of decreased ventricular compliance.

Initial Diagnostic Results: His 12-lead EKG shows ST depression in leads V2-V6 and leads I and aVL, with T-wave inversions in the lateral leads. These changes are new compared to his baseline EKG from six months ago. Initial troponin I is 0.12 ng/mL (elevated, suggesting myocardial injury), and chest X-ray shows mild pulmonary vascular congestion.

Risk Stratification Assessment: Mr. Chen's presentation meets criteria for high-risk unstable angina based on multiple factors including ongoing chest pain despite medical therapy, new EKG changes, elevated cardiac biomarkers, and his extensive history of coronary disease. The TIMI (Thrombolysis in Myocardial Infarction) risk score helps quantify his short-term risk of adverse cardiac events.

TIMI Risk Score Calculation:

- Age ≥65 years: 1 point (he's 68)

- ≥3 CAD risk factors: 1 point (diabetes, hypertension, hyperlipidemia, family history)

- Known CAD with stenosis ≥50%: 1 point (documented multivessel disease)

- Aspirin use within 7 days: 1 point (on chronic therapy)

- Severe angina (≥2 episodes within 24 hours): 1 point (current prolonged episode)

- EKG changes: 1 point (new ST depressions)

- Elevated cardiac markers: 1 point (troponin 0.12 ng/mL)

Total TIMI Score: 7 points (indicating very high risk with >40% probability of death, MI, or urgent revascularization within 14 days)

NGN-Style Bowtie with Multiple Pathways:

Central Problem: 68-year-old with high-risk unstable angina and multi-vessel coronary disease

Assessment Parameters (Select all appropriate):

- Serial cardiac enzymes every 6-8 hours
- Continuous cardiac monitoring for arrhythmias
- Frequent vital signs and pain assessments
- Echocardiogram to assess wall motion abnormalities
- Chest X-ray to evaluate for pulmonary edema
- Preparation for urgent cardiac catheterization

Immediate Interventions (Select treatment pathway):

Pathway A - Conservative Medical Management:

- Optimize antianginal medications
- Increase beta-blocker and add nitrates
- Schedule elective catheterization within 72 hours
- Monitor for symptom resolution

Pathway B - Urgent Invasive Strategy:

- Emergent cardiac catheterization within 2 hours
- Activate interventional cardiology team
- Prepare for possible multi-vessel intervention
- Consider surgical consultation for complex disease

Pathway C - Intermediate Strategy:

- Admit to coronary care unit for observation

- Optimize medical therapy for 24-48 hours

- Schedule urgent catheterization if symptoms persist

- Monitor troponin trend and EKG changes

Correct Pathway Selection: Pathway B (Urgent Invasive Strategy)

Rationale: TIMI score of 7 indicates very high-risk unstable angina requiring urgent invasive management. His ongoing symptoms despite medical therapy, new EKG changes, and elevated biomarkers make conservative management inappropriate. Early invasive strategy (within 24 hours, preferably within 2 hours) improves outcomes in high-risk patients (76).

Urgent Invasive Management Protocol

Pre-Catheterization Preparation: Mr. Chen receives aggressive medical therapy while preparing for emergent catheterization. This includes intravenous heparin, optimization of antiplatelet therapy, and careful hemodynamic monitoring. The interventional cardiology team is activated, and the catheterization laboratory is prepared for complex multi-vessel intervention.

Catheterization Findings: Cardiac catheterization reveals severe three-vessel coronary disease with 95% stenosis in the proximal left anterior descending artery (LAD), 85% stenosis in the circumflex artery, and 80% stenosis in the right coronary artery (site of previous stent). The left ventricular ejection fraction is 45%, indicating mild systolic dysfunction.

Revascularization Decision-Making: The interventional cardiologist, cardiac surgeon, and heart team discuss options for revascularization. Given the complexity of his disease, significant comorbidities, and patient preferences, they must choose between percutaneous coronary intervention (PCI) and coronary artery bypass grafting (CABG).

Treatment Options Analysis:

Option 1 - Staged PCI: Treat the culprit LAD lesion immediately, then address other vessels in subsequent procedures

- **Advantages**: Less invasive, faster recovery, addresses immediate threat
- **Disadvantages**: May require multiple procedures, incomplete revascularization initially

Option 2 - Complete PCI: Attempt to treat all significant lesions in single procedure

- **Advantages**: Complete revascularization, single procedure
- **Disadvantages**: Increased contrast load, longer procedure time, technical complexity

Option 3 - CABG: Surgical revascularization with bypass grafts to all affected vessels

- **Advantages**: Most complete revascularization, better long-term outcomes for complex disease
- **Disadvantages**: More invasive, longer recovery, higher immediate risk

Case Resolution: The heart team decides on staged PCI, beginning with intervention on the culprit LAD lesion. The proximal LAD stenosis is successfully treated with a drug-eluting stent, resulting in excellent angiographic result and resolution of Mr. Chen's chest pain. Plans are made for staged intervention on the circumflex artery within 4-6 weeks, with the right coronary artery lesion to be managed medically given its location within the previous stent.

Scenario 38: Post-Cardiac Surgery Complications

Patient Background: Margaret Washington, a 70-year-old retired librarian, is 48 hours post-operative following coronary artery bypass grafting (CABG) with three vessel bypasses. Her surgery was technically successful, but she's developed concerning signs that suggest possible cardiac tamponade—a life-threatening complication that requires immediate recognition and intervention. The cardiac surgery team is monitoring her closely, but early signs can be subtle and easily missed without careful assessment.

Mrs. Washington's surgery involved bypasses to the LAD, circumflex, and right coronary arteries using both internal mammary artery and saphenous vein grafts. Her initial post-operative course was unremarkable, and she was extubated on post-operative day one. However, over the past 12 hours, her nursing team has noticed gradual changes in her hemodynamic status that individually seem minor but collectively suggest developing complications (77).

Current Clinical Status: Mrs. Washington appears comfortable but somewhat fatigued. She's been asking for more pain medication despite her incisions appearing well-healed and showing no signs of infection. Her family reports that she seems "not quite herself" and appears more tired than expected for this stage of recovery.

Hemodynamic Assessment: Her vital signs show subtle but concerning trends: blood pressure has decreased from 125/70 to 105/65 over the past 8 hours, heart rate has increased from 80 to 100 bpm, and she's developed a paradoxical pulse (pulsus paradoxus) of 12 mmHg. Central venous pressure has risen from 8 to 14 mmHg, and her urine output has decreased to 25 mL/hr over the past 4 hours.

Physical Examination Findings: Cardiac examination reveals distant heart sounds, elevated jugular venous pressure, and the presence of pulsus paradoxus. Her chest tube drainage has decreased significantly over the past 24 hours (from 200 mL/shift to 50 mL/shift), which might initially seem reassuring but could indicate tube occlusion rather than decreased bleeding.

NGN-Style Matrix for Complication Recognition:

Categorize the following assessment findings as "High Suspicion for Tamponade," "Moderate Concern," or "Normal Post-Operative Finding":

Hemodynamic Parameters:

- Paradoxical pulse 12 mmHg: High Suspicion for Tamponade

- Central venous pressure 14 mmHg: High Suspicion for Tamponade

- Blood pressure decrease from 125/70 to 105/65: Moderate Concern

- Heart rate increase from 80 to 100: Moderate Concern

- Urine output 25 mL/hr for 4 hours: High Suspicion for Tamponade

Physical Assessment:

- Distant heart sounds: High Suspicion for Tamponade

- Elevated jugular venous distension: High Suspicion for Tamponade

- Decreased chest tube drainage: High Suspicion for Tamponade

- Patient reports of fatigue: Moderate Concern

- Well-healed surgical incisions: Normal Post-Operative Finding

Clinical Presentation:

- Increased pain medication requests: Moderate Concern

- Family reports patient "not quite herself": Moderate Concern

- Comfortable appearance at rest: Normal Post-Operative Finding

Rationale: Cardiac tamponade presents with Beck's triad (elevated JVP, hypotension, distant heart sounds) plus pulsus paradoxus. The combination of hemodynamic changes, decreased chest tube output, and clinical symptoms creates high suspicion requiring immediate intervention (78).

Emergency Assessment and Intervention

Immediate Diagnostic Confirmation: The cardiac surgery team orders an urgent echocardiogram to confirm the diagnosis of cardiac tamponade. The study shows a moderate pericardial effusion with evidence of right atrial and right ventricular diastolic collapse, confirming hemodynamically significant tamponade.

Emergency Intervention Protocol: Cardiac tamponade requires immediate surgical intervention to relieve the pressure around the heart. Mrs. Washington is taken emergently to the operating room for pericardial window or surgical exploration to evacuate the accumulated blood and fluid compressing her heart.

Pre-Operative Preparation:

1. **Hemodynamic support**: Fluid resuscitation to maintain preload while avoiding excessive volume

2. **Anesthesia considerations**: Careful induction to prevent cardiovascular collapse

3. **Surgical team activation**: Immediate availability of cardiac surgeon and perfusionist

4. **Family communication**: Urgent discussion about the complication and need for emergency surgery

Intraoperative Findings: During surgical exploration, the team discovers approximately 400 mL of blood and clot in the pericardial space compressing the heart. No active bleeding source is identified, suggesting the tamponade resulted from gradual accumulation of blood that failed to drain through the chest tubes, possibly due to clot formation.

Post-Intervention Recovery: Following evacuation of the pericardial fluid and placement of additional drainage tubes, Mrs. Washington's hemodynamic status improves dramatically. Her blood pressure returns to 120/75, heart rate decreases to 85 bpm, central venous pressure normalizes to 8 mmHg, and urine output increases to normal levels.

Recognition Patterns for Post-Cardiac Surgery Complications

Early Warning Signs: Successful management of post-cardiac surgery complications depends on early recognition of subtle changes that precede obvious clinical deterioration. Nurses caring for cardiac surgery patients must maintain high vigilance for signs of bleeding, tamponade, low cardiac output syndrome, and arrhythmias.

Common Post-Operative Complications:

Bleeding and Tamponade:

- Monitor chest tube output quantity and quality

- Assess for signs of cardiac compression

- Watch for hemodynamic changes suggesting volume loss or cardiac compression

Low Cardiac Output Syndrome:

- Monitor urine output as early indicator of cardiac output

- Assess perfusion indicators (skin temperature, capillary refill, mental status)

- Watch for signs of cardiogenic shock

Arrhythmias:

- Continuous cardiac monitoring for first 48-72 hours

- Electrolyte monitoring and correction

- Recognition of life-threatening rhythm disturbances

Infection:

- Monitor for signs of surgical site infection or mediastinitis

- Temperature trends and white blood cell count monitoring

- Assessment of wound healing and drainage

Clinical Decision-Making in Complex Cardiac Care

These advanced cardiac scenarios demonstrate the sophisticated clinical reasoning required for complex cardiovascular nursing. Both cases involve rapid assessment, risk stratification, and coordination of multiple interventions while maintaining focus on patient safety and optimal outcomes.

Risk Assessment Skills: Understanding how to use validated risk stratification tools like the TIMI score helps quantify patient risk and guide treatment intensity. These tools supplement but don't replace clinical judgment in determining appropriate interventions.

Complication Recognition: Post-operative cardiac patients require skilled nursing assessment to detect early signs of life-threatening complications. The ability to recognize subtle changes that indicate developing problems can mean the difference between routine recovery and emergency intervention.

Interdisciplinary Collaboration: Complex cardiac care requires seamless coordination between nursing, cardiology, cardiac surgery, and other specialties. Effective communication and shared decision-making optimize patient outcomes while ensuring all team members understand their roles and responsibilities.

Professional Development Through Complex Cases

These scenarios prepare you for advanced cardiovascular nursing practice where patients present with multiple comorbidities, complex decision-making requirements, and potential for rapid clinical deterioration. The integration of assessment skills, clinical reasoning, and intervention coordination represents the highest level of nursing expertise.

Each case builds upon foundational knowledge while introducing concepts about advanced cardiac pathophysiology, complex therapeutic interventions, and professional responsibilities. The emphasis on early recognition, rapid intervention, and interdisciplinary communication reflects the reality that cardiovascular nursing often involves life-and-death decisions made under pressure.

Clinical Excellence and Patient Advocacy

Advanced cardiac scenarios remind us that nursing expertise extends beyond technical skills to include advocacy for appropriate care, support for patients and families during stressful situations, and commitment to continuous learning and professional development. Your role involves not just implementing interventions but ensuring that patients receive the right care at the right time while maintaining their dignity and involvement in decision-making.

The complexity of these cases reflects the reality of modern cardiovascular care, where patients live longer with more complex conditions requiring sophisticated nursing expertise and interdisciplinary coordination. The knowledge and skills you develop through engaging with these scenarios will serve you throughout your career as cardiovascular nursing continues to evolve with advancing technology and changing patient populations.

Wisdom in Practice

These complex cardiac scenarios serve as more than educational exercises—they represent the daily reality faced by cardiovascular nurses who must think quickly, act decisively, and coordinate care for patients whose conditions can change in moments. Each case teaches us that expertise comes not just from knowledge but from the wisdom to apply that knowledge appropriately in dynamic, high-stakes situations.

The progression from recognizing unstable angina requiring urgent intervention to identifying post-operative complications demanding immediate surgery illustrates how nursing practice evolves from following protocols to making sophisticated clinical judgments. This journey represents the heart of professional nursing development— the transformation from competent practitioner to expert clinician capable of leading complex care initiatives.

Your engagement with these scenarios prepares you not just for examinations or clinical rotations, but for a career of continuous learning, professional growth, and service to patients and families during some of their most vulnerable moments. The expertise you develop will ripple outward, influencing not only your own practice but the development of colleagues and the quality of care provided by your healthcare teams.

Key Learning Points

- Multi-vessel coronary disease requires risk stratification using validated tools like the TIMI score

- High-risk unstable angina warrants urgent invasive strategy rather than conservative management

- Cardiac tamponade presents with subtle early signs requiring high clinical suspicion

- Post-operative complications demand continuous vigilance and early intervention capabilities

- Complex cardiac care requires seamless interdisciplinary collaboration and communication

- Risk assessment tools supplement but don't replace clinical judgment in treatment decisions

- Early recognition of complications prevents progression to life-threatening situations

- Family communication during cardiac emergencies requires honesty balanced with appropriate hope

- Advanced cardiac nursing integrates technical expertise with sophisticated clinical reasoning

- Professional development in cardiovascular care requires commitment to lifelong learning and continuous improvement

Chapter 16: Advanced Critical Care and Emergency Scenarios

The intersection of clinical expertise, leadership skills, and ethical reasoning defines the highest levels of nursing practice. These advanced scenarios place you at the center of complex medical emergencies and ethical dilemmas where split-second decisions can determine patient outcomes and where your professional judgment shapes not only individual care but entire healthcare team responses. From managing multiple organ failure to leading disaster response efforts, these situations demand the full spectrum of nursing knowledge and professional competency.

Scenario 39: Septic Shock with Multiple Organ Dysfunction Syndrome (MODS)

Patient Background: Michael Rodriguez, a 55-year-old maintenance supervisor, presents to the intensive care unit with severe urosepsis that has progressed to septic shock with multiple organ dysfunction syndrome. He initially sought care at his primary physician's office three days ago with urinary frequency and burning, but his condition rapidly deteriorated despite oral antibiotic therapy. His wife brought him to the emergency department this morning when she found him confused, hypotensive, and barely responsive.

Mr. Rodriguez has a history of benign prostatic hyperplasia, diabetes mellitus type 2 (well-controlled), and mild chronic kidney disease. He underwent prostate biopsy two weeks ago for elevated PSA levels, which may have introduced bacteria into his urinary system. His infection has now progressed to involve multiple organ systems, requiring aggressive intervention and continuous monitoring across all body systems (70).

Current Clinical Status: Mr. Rodriguez is intubated and mechanically ventilated due to respiratory failure and altered mental status. He requires continuous renal replacement therapy for acute kidney injury and multiple vasoactive medications to maintain blood pressure. His condition represents the most severe form of sepsis, with evidence of dysfunction in respiratory, cardiovascular, renal, neurological, and hematological systems.

Organ System Assessment:

- **Respiratory**: Acute respiratory distress syndrome with bilateral infiltrates, requiring high PEEP and FiO2

- **Cardiovascular**: Distributive shock requiring norepinephrine, vasopressin, and epinephrine

- **Renal**: Acute kidney injury with anuria, requiring continuous venovenous hemofiltration

- **Neurological**: Encephalopathy with Glasgow Coma Scale of 6, no response to verbal stimuli

- **Hematological**: Disseminated intravascular coagulation with low platelets and elevated D-dimer

- **Hepatic**: Elevated liver enzymes and bilirubin indicating hepatic dysfunction

Sepsis Bundle Compliance Assessment: The Surviving Sepsis Campaign guidelines require specific interventions within defined timeframes to optimize outcomes. Mr. Rodriguez's care is evaluated against these evidence-based benchmarks to ensure all appropriate interventions are implemented promptly and effectively.

NGN-Style Unfolding Case with Multiple Systems:

Hour 1 - Initial ICU Management:

Surviving Sepsis Campaign Bundle Components (Assess completion status):

1. **Blood cultures obtained before antibiotics**: Completed in ED before broad-spectrum antibiotics

2. **Lactate measurement**: Initial lactate 6.8 mmol/L, indicating severe tissue hypoperfusion

3. **Broad-spectrum antibiotics**: Piperacillin-tazobactam and vancomycin initiated within 1 hour

4. **Fluid resuscitation**: 30 mL/kg crystalloid completed (2.1 L for 70 kg patient)

5. **Vasopressors for persistent hypotension**: Norepinephrine initiated for MAP <65 mmHg

6. **Source control**: Urology consultation for possible drainage procedure

Hour 6 - Ongoing Management and Assessment: Despite initial bundle compliance, Mr. Rodriguez shows signs of worsening organ dysfunction. His lactate has increased to 8.2 mmol/L, urine output remains minimal despite fluid resuscitation, and ventilator requirements have increased due to worsening ARDS.

Multi-System Support Strategies:

Respiratory Support:

- Mechanical ventilation with lung-protective strategy (6 mL/kg tidal volume)

- PEEP optimization to improve oxygenation while minimizing barotrauma

- Prone positioning protocol if P/F ratio remains below 150

- Sedation management to facilitate ventilator synchrony

Cardiovascular Support:

- Titrate vasopressors to maintain MAP 65-70 mmHg

- Monitor cardiac output and systemic vascular resistance

- Consider adding vasopressin or epinephrine for refractory shock

- Evaluate for myocardial depression with echocardiography

Renal Support:

- Continuous renal replacement therapy for fluid and electrolyte management

- Monitor for electrolyte imbalances and acid-base disturbances

- Adjust medication doses for renal replacement therapy

- Assess daily for recovery of renal function

Hour 24 - Critical Decision Points: Mr. Rodriguez shows mixed response to treatment. His lactate has decreased to 4.1 mmol/L (indicating some improvement in tissue perfusion), but he's developed new complications including gastrointestinal bleeding and further deterioration in liver function.

Prognostic Assessment Tools:

- **APACHE II score**: 28 points (predicted mortality 55-75%)

- **SOFA score**: 15 points (indicating severe organ dysfunction)

- **Sepsis-related organ failure assessment**: Involvement of 4 organ systems

Family Communication and Goals of Care: The healthcare team meets with Mr. Rodriguez's wife and adult children to discuss his condition, prognosis, and treatment options. This conversation requires balancing honest prognostic information with hope while exploring the family's understanding of his values and wishes for care.

Scenario 40: Acute Respiratory Distress Syndrome (ARDS) Management

Patient Background: Sandra Martinez, a 48-year-old emergency department nurse, develops severe ARDS following aspiration pneumonia that occurred during a complicated intubation for emergency surgery. As a healthcare worker, she understands the severity of her condition, which adds psychological complexity to her care. Her illness began five days ago with what seemed like a minor

174

surgical procedure, but aspiration during induction led to rapidly progressive respiratory failure.

Ms. Martinez has no significant past medical history and was previously healthy and active. The irony of her situation—being cared for by colleagues in the same hospital where she works—creates unique challenges for both the patient and her caregivers. Her husband and teenage children are struggling with seeing her in such a vulnerable state, especially given her role as a healthcare provider (71).

Current Respiratory Status: Ms. Martinez requires mechanical ventilation with high oxygen requirements and positive end-expiratory pressure (PEEP). Her chest X-rays show bilateral infiltrates consistent with ARDS, and her oxygenation index indicates severe disease. She's alert and follows commands, which creates additional challenges as she's aware of every intervention and complication.

ARDS Severity Classification:

- **PaO2/FiO2 ratio**: 85 mmHg (severe ARDS, normal >300)

- **PEEP requirement**: 15 cm H2O to maintain adequate oxygenation

- **Chest imaging**: Bilateral infiltrates in all lung fields

- **Clinical course**: Rapid onset following known risk factor (aspiration)

Ventilator Management Protocol: Evidence-based ARDS management requires specific ventilator strategies to minimize ventilator-induced lung injury while maintaining adequate gas exchange. The ARDSNet protocol guides ventilator settings and adjustment criteria.

NGN-Style Trend Analysis with Interventions:

Day 1 - Initial ARDS Management:

- **Tidal volume**: 6 mL/kg predicted body weight (420 mL for her 70 kg frame)

- **PEEP**: Starting at 12 cm H2O, titrated based on oxygenation and compliance

- **FiO2**: 0.8 initially, goal to reduce below 0.6 to prevent oxygen toxicity

- **Plateau pressure**: Maintain below 30 cm H2O to prevent barotrauma

Day 3 - Worsening Oxygenation: Despite optimal ventilator management, Ms. Martinez's oxygenation deteriorates. Her P/F ratio drops to 65 mmHg, indicating severe, refractory ARDS requiring consideration of rescue therapies.

Advanced ARDS Interventions:

Prone Positioning Protocol:

1. **Criteria assessment**: P/F ratio <150 on FiO2 ≥0.6 and PEEP ≥5 cm H2O

2. **Team preparation**: Minimum 5 trained staff members for safe positioning

3. **Duration**: 16-hour prone sessions with 8-hour supine periods

4. **Monitoring**: Continuous assessment for complications (pressure injuries, tube displacement)

Neuromuscular Blockade:

- **Indication**: Severe ARDS with ventilator dyssynchrony despite deep sedation

- **Agent**: Cisatracurium infusion for 48 hours maximum

- **Monitoring**: Train-of-four monitoring to prevent over-paralysis

- **Complications**: Weakness, critical illness myopathy prevention

Day 5 - Prone Positioning Response: After 48 hours of prone positioning cycles, Ms. Martinez shows improved oxygenation. Her P/F ratio increases to 120 mmHg, allowing reduction in FiO2 from 0.8 to 0.65. The improvement indicates beneficial effects of prone positioning on ventilation-perfusion matching.

Recovery Phase Management:

- Gradual weaning of PEEP and FiO2 as oxygenation improves

- Daily spontaneous breathing trials to assess readiness for extubation

- Prevention of ventilator-associated complications (pneumonia, delirium)

- Physical therapy to prevent ICU-acquired weakness

Scenario 41: Hepatorenal Syndrome

Patient Presentation

James Martinez, 58-year-old male

Background: History of alcoholic cirrhosis (Child-Pugh Class C), admitted 3 days ago with acute decompensation. Has developed progressive oliguria despite initial diuretic therapy being held.

Current Status - Day 3, 0800:

- Alert but lethargic, oriented x2 (person, place)

- Massive ascites with tense, distended abdomen

- 3+ pitting edema to mid-thigh bilaterally

- Jaundiced with scleral icterus

- No asterixis currently noted

Vital Signs:

- BP: 88/52 mmHg (MAP 64)

- HR: 110 bpm, regular

- RR: 24/min, shallow due to abdominal distension

- Temp: 98.8°F (37.1°C)

- O2 sat: 92% on 2L nasal cannula

- Weight: 89 kg (up 12 kg from baseline dry weight of 77 kg)

Laboratory Results:

Test	Current (Day 3)	Previous (Day 1)	Normal Range
Creatinine	2.8 mg/dL	1.4 mg/dL	0.7-1.3 mg/dL
BUN	68 mg/dL	32 mg/dL	7-20 mg/dL
Sodium	128 mEq/L	134 mEq/L	136-145 mEq/L
Potassium	5.2 mEq/L	4.1 mEq/L	3.5-5.0 mEq/L
Albumin	2.1 g/dL	2.2 g/dL	3.5-5.0 g/dL
Total Bilirubin	8.4 mg/dL	6.2 mg/dL	0.3-1.2 mg/dL
INR	2.8	2.4	0.8-1.1
Urine Output	180 mL/24hr	400 mL/24hr	>800 mL/24hr

Additional Findings:

- Urine sodium: 8 mEq/L (suggests prerenal etiology)

- Fractional excretion of sodium (FENa): 0.3%

- No evidence of nephrotoxic medications

- Renal ultrasound: Normal size kidneys, no obstruction

- Recent paracentesis removed 4L fluid with appropriate albumin replacement

---

NGN Matrix Question: Competing Priorities in Hepatorenal Syndrome

Instructions: For each clinical priority below, select ALL interventions that are appropriate. Each priority may have multiple correct interventions, and interventions may be used for multiple priorities.

Clinical Priorities:

A. Optimize Renal Perfusion B. Manage Fluid Overload
C. Prevent Further Hepatic Decompensation D. Monitor for Complications

Available Interventions:

1. Administer octreotide 50 mcg subcutaneous q8h

2. Initiate continuous renal replacement therapy (CRRT)

3. Give furosemide 80 mg IV push

4. Administer albumin 25% 100 mL IV

5. Prepare for large-volume paracentesis

6. Start midodrine 7.5 mg PO q8h

7. Restrict sodium to <2g/day

8. Monitor daily weights and strict I&O

9. Hold ACE inhibitors and diuretics

10. Obtain hepatology consultation for TIPS evaluation

11. Check electrolytes q6h

12. Position patient in semi-Fowler's with legs elevated

13. Administer norepinephrine if MAP <65 mmHg

14. Restrict fluid intake to <1.5L/day

15. Monitor for hepatic encephalopathy signs

Matrix Answer Key:

Intervention	A. Optimize Renal Perfusion	B. Manage Fluid Overload	C. Prevent Hepatic Decompensation	D. Monitor for Complications
1. Octreotide	✓			
2. CRRT		✓		
3. Furosemide		X (contraindicated)		
4. Albumin 25%	✓		✓	
5. Large-volume paracentesis		✓		
6. Midodrine	✓			
7. Sodium restriction		✓	✓	
8. Daily weights/I&O		✓		✓

Intervention	A. Optimize Renal Perfusion	B. Manage Fluid Overload	C. Prevent Hepatic Decompensation	D. Monitor for Complications
9. Hold ACE inhibitors/diuretics	✓			
10. Hepatology consult/TIPS	✓	✓	✓	
11. Electrolytes q6h				✓
12. Semi-Fowler's position		✓		
13. Norepinephrine	✓			
14. Fluid restriction		✓		
15. Monitor encephalopathy			✓	✓

Rationales:

Priority A - Optimize Renal Perfusion:

- **Octreotide:** Reduces splanchnic vasodilation, improving systemic vascular resistance

- **Albumin:** Expands intravascular volume and improves oncotic pressure

- **Midodrine:** Alpha-agonist that increases systemic vascular resistance

- **Hold ACE inhibitors/diuretics:** Prevents further reduction in renal perfusion pressure

- **Norepinephrine:** Vasopressor support if MAP <65 mmHg despite other measures

- **TIPS evaluation:** Definitive treatment by reducing portal pressure

Priority B - Manage Fluid Overload:

- **CRRT:** For fluid removal when diuretics contraindicated

- **Large-volume paracentesis:** Removes ascitic fluid, improves breathing and comfort

- **Sodium/fluid restrictions:** Prevents further fluid accumulation

- **Daily weights/I&O:** Monitors fluid balance trends

- **Semi-Fowler's positioning:** Facilitates breathing with ascites

- **TIPS:** Reduces ascites formation by decreasing portal pressure

Priority C - Prevent Further Hepatic Decompensation:

- **Albumin:** Maintains oncotic pressure, supports liver function

- **Sodium restriction:** Reduces ascites formation

- **Monitor encephalopathy:** Early detection of worsening liver function

- **TIPS:** May improve overall hepatic function by reducing portal hypertension

Priority D - Monitor for Complications:

- **Daily weights/I&O:** Tracks fluid balance and treatment response

- **Electrolytes q6h:** Monitors for dangerous electrolyte shifts

- **Monitor encephalopathy:** Critical complication requiring immediate intervention

Key Learning Points:

1. Hepatorenal syndrome requires balancing competing priorities of fluid management

2. Traditional diuretics are contraindicated as they worsen renal perfusion

3. The combination of octreotide, midodrine, and albumin is first-line therapy

4. TIPS may be both therapeutic and diagnostic for treatment-resistant cases

5. Careful monitoring prevents life-threatening complications during treatment

---

Scenario 42: Severe Pancreatitis

Initial Presentation - Emergency Department

Maria Rodriguez, 45-year-old female

Chief Complaint: "The worst abdominal pain of my life - it started yesterday and keeps getting worse."

History of Present Illness: Patient reports sudden onset of severe epigastric pain 36 hours ago that radiates to her back. Pain is constant, 10/10 intensity, worse when lying flat, partially relieved by leaning forward. Associated with nausea, vomiting (unable to keep anything down), and fever. Denies alcohol use but admits to recent gallbladder "attacks" over past 6 months that she ignored.

Past Medical History:

- Cholelithiasis (known but untreated)
- Hypertension
- Type 2 diabetes (well-controlled)
- No previous hospitalizations

Current Vital Signs:

- BP: 92/58 mmHg
- HR: 118 bpm, regular
- RR: 28/min, shallow
- Temp: 101.8°F (38.8°C)
- O2 sat: 94% on room air
- Pain: 10/10 epigastric

Physical Assessment:

- Appears acutely ill, diaphoretic, restless with pain
- Abdomen: Severely tender epigastrium with guarding, hypoactive bowel sounds
- Positive Cullen's sign (periumbilical ecchymosis)
- Positive Grey Turner's sign (flank ecchymosis)
- No palpable masses, no rebound tenderness
- Lungs: Bilateral fine crackles in bases
- Heart: Tachycardic, regular rhythm

Phase 1: Emergency Department Assessment (Hour 0-2)

Initial Laboratory Results:

Test	Result	Normal Range
Lipase	2,840 U/L	10-140 U/L
Amylase	1,200 U/L	30-110 U/L
WBC	18,500/μL	4,000-11,000/μL
Hgb/Hct	14.2 g/dL / 42%	12-16 g/dL / 36-46%
Platelets	280,000/μL	150-450,000/μL
Glucose	245 mg/dL	70-100 mg/dL
Calcium	7.8 mg/dL	8.5-10.5 mg/dL
BUN/Creatinine	28/1.4 mg/dL	7-20 / 0.7-1.3 mg/dL
ALT/AST	156/198 U/L	7-35 / 8-40 U/L
Total Bilirubin	3.2 mg/dL	0.3-1.2 mg/dL
Lactate	3.8 mmol/L	0.5-2.2 mmol/L

Imaging Results:

CT Abdomen with Contrast:

- Pancreatic enlargement with heterogeneous enhancement
- Peripancreatic fluid collections
- Gallbladder wall thickening with multiple stones
- No evidence of pancreatic necrosis at this time
- Small bilateral pleural effusions

NGN Question 1: Initial Priority Actions

Select the 3 highest priority interventions for this patient in the first 2 hours:

A. Obtain surgical consultation for immediate cholecystectomy B. Initiate aggressive IV fluid resuscitation with lactated Ringer's C. Administer morphine 4 mg IV every 2 hours for pain control D. Begin enteral nutrition within 6 hours E. Insert nasogastric tube for gastric decompression F. Administer broad-spectrum antibiotics G. Monitor urine output and consider Foley catheter H. Prepare for endoscopic retrograde cholangiopancreatography (ERCP)

Phase 2: ICU Admission - Day 1 (Hour 12-24)

Patient Status Update: Despite initial resuscitation, patient's condition has deteriorated. Transferred to ICU for closer monitoring.

Current Vital Signs:

- BP: 85/48 mmHg (on 500 mL fluid bolus)

- HR: 132 bpm

- RR: 32/min

- Temp: 102.4°F (39.1°C)

- O2 sat: 89% on 4L nasal cannula

- Urine output: 15 mL/hr for past 4 hours

Updated Laboratory Results (24 hours):

Test	Hour 0	Hour 24	Trend
Lipase	2,840 U/L	3,200 U/L	↑
WBC	18,500/μL	22,000/μL	↑

Test	Hour 0	Hour 24	Trend
Hgb/Hct	14.2/42%	16.8/50%	↑ (hemoconcentration)
Calcium	7.8 mg/dL	6.9 mg/dL	↓
Creatinine	1.4 mg/dL	2.1 mg/dL	↑
Lactate	3.8 mmol/L	5.2 mmol/L	↑

New Findings:

- Developing acute respiratory distress with bilateral infiltrates on chest X-ray

- Oliguria despite adequate fluid resuscitation

- Patient becoming more lethargic, oriented only to name

NGN Question 2: Recognizing Complications

Which complications is this patient most likely developing? Select ALL that apply:

A. Acute respiratory distress syndrome (ARDS) B. Acute kidney injury (AKI) C. Hypocalcemic tetany D. Pancreatic pseudocyst E. Systemic inflammatory response syndrome (SIRS) F. Infected pancreatic necrosis G. Splenic vein thrombosis H. Diabetes mellitus

NGN Question 3: Revised Treatment Priorities

Based on the patient's deterioration, rank these interventions in order of priority (1 = highest priority):

___ Initiate continuous renal replacement therapy (CRRT) ___ Begin mechanical ventilation with lung-protective strategies ___ Administer calcium gluconate for symptomatic hypocalcemia ___ Start vasopressor support (norepinephrine) ___ Obtain repeat CT scan to assess for pancreatic necrosis ___ Begin parenteral nutrition ___ Insert central venous catheter for monitoring ___ Consult interventional radiology for possible drainage

Phase 3: Day 3-5 - Stabilization and Nutrition Focus

Patient Status Update: Patient has been stabilized on mechanical ventilation and vasopressors. Now focusing on nutritional support and preventing further complications.

Current Status:

- Intubated and sedated, hemodynamically stable on low-dose norepinephrine

- Urine output improved to 40 mL/hr with CRRT support

- Repeat CT shows 30% pancreatic necrosis, no definite infection

Nutrition Assessment:

- NPO for 72 hours

- Pre-illness weight: 68 kg

- Current weight: 74 kg (fluid retention)

- Albumin: 2.4 g/dL

- Prealbumin: 12 mg/dL (normal 15-36 mg/dL)

NGN Question 4: Nutritional Management Decision Tree

The patient has been NPO for 72 hours. What is the most appropriate nutritional approach?

If the patient has minimal nausea and bowel sounds are present: A. Continue NPO and reassess in 24 hours B. Begin clear liquids and advance as tolerated C. Start enteral nutrition via nasojejunal tube D. Initiate parenteral nutrition immediately

If the patient has persistent ileus and absent bowel sounds: A. Wait for return of bowel function before any nutrition B. Begin parenteral nutrition within 48 hours C. Start enteral nutrition via nasogastric tube D. Continue NPO with IV dextrose only

If enteral nutrition is not tolerated after 48 hours: A. Return to NPO status B. Reduce enteral rate and add prokinetic agents C. Switch to parenteral nutrition D. Try different enteral formula

NGN Question 5: Pain Management Strategy

The patient is now awake and extubated but experiencing severe pain (8/10). Select the BEST multimodal pain management approach:

Primary analgesics (select 2): A. Morphine PCA 1 mg q10min, 10 mg 4-hour lockout B. Fentanyl continuous infusion 25 mcg/hr C. Hydromorphone PCA 0.2 mg q10min, 2 mg 4-hour lockout D. Meperidine 50 mg IM q4h PRN

Adjunctive therapies (select 2): A. Acetaminophen 1000 mg q6h (if no hepatic concerns) B. Ketorolac 30 mg IV q6h C. Gabapentin 300 mg TID D. Celecoxib 200 mg BID

Non-pharmacological interventions (select 2): A. Heat application to abdomen B. Positioning in semi-Fowler's with knees flexed C. TENS unit application D. Deep breathing and relaxation techniques

---

Phase 4: Day 7-10 - Recovery and Discharge Planning

Patient Status: Patient has shown significant improvement. Off mechanical ventilation, vasopressors discontinued, kidney function recovering.

Current Issues:

- Tolerating enteral nutrition at goal rate

- Pain controlled with oral medications

- Concern about pancreatic enzyme insufficiency

- Planning for long-term management

NGN Question 6: Discharge Planning Priorities

Prioritize these discharge planning elements (1 = most important):

___ Pancreatic enzyme replacement therapy education ___ Diabetes management and glucose monitoring ___ Alcohol cessation counseling (even though patient denies use) ___ Follow-up imaging schedule to monitor pseudocyst development ___ Cholecystectomy planning once inflammation resolves ___ Dietary counseling for low-fat, small frequent meals ___ Recognition of signs/symptoms requiring immediate medical attention ___ Gradual return to normal activities timeline

---

Answer Keys and Rationales

Phase 1 Answer:

Correct selections: B, G, H

- **B. IV fluid resuscitation:** Critical for preventing pancreatic ischemia and organ failure

- **G. Monitor urine output:** Essential for assessing adequacy of resuscitation

- **H. ERCP:** Indicated for gallstone pancreatitis with evidence of biliary obstruction

Phase 2 Complications Answer:

Correct selections: A, B, C, E

- Patient showing signs of multi-organ dysfunction syndrome

Phase 2 Priority Ranking:

1. **Begin mechanical ventilation** (respiratory failure is immediately life-threatening)

2. **Start vasopressor support** (hemodynamic instability)

3. **Administer calcium gluconate** (symptomatic hypocalcemia can cause cardiac issues)

4. **Insert central venous catheter** (needed for vasopressors and monitoring)

5. **Initiate CRRT** (acute kidney injury management)

6. **Obtain repeat CT scan** (assess for complications)

7. **Consult interventional radiology** (if infected necrosis suspected)

8. **Begin parenteral nutrition** (not immediate priority)

Nutrition Decision Tree Answers:

- **With bowel sounds present:** C. Start enteral nutrition via nasojejunal tube

- **With persistent ileus:** B. Begin parenteral nutrition within 48 hours

- **If enteral not tolerated:** C. Switch to parenteral nutrition

Pain Management Answer:

Primary analgesics: A and C (PCA allows patient control while providing adequate analgesia) **Adjunctive therapies:** A and C (acetaminophen and gabapentin are safe additions) **Non-pharmacological:** B and D (positioning and relaxation techniques are helpful)

Discharge Planning Priority Order:

1. Recognition of signs/symptoms requiring immediate medical attention

2. Cholecystectomy planning once inflammation resolves

3. Pancreatic enzyme replacement therapy education

4. Dietary counseling for low-fat, small frequent meals

5. Follow-up imaging schedule to monitor pseudocyst development

6. Diabetes management and glucose monitoring

7. Gradual return to normal activities timeline

8. Alcohol cessation counseling

Key Learning Points:

- Severe pancreatitis requires aggressive early resuscitation

- Multi-organ dysfunction can develop rapidly

- Early enteral nutrition is preferred when tolerated

- Pain management requires multimodal approach

- Long-term complications require ongoing monitoring and management

Chapter 17: Emergency and Leadership Scenarios

Scenario 43: Code Blue Leadership

Patient Background: Eleanor Washington, a 65-year-old retired teacher, was admitted to the medical unit two days ago with pneumonia and has been responding well to antibiotic therapy. However, at 1430, her nurse finds her unresponsive in bed during routine medication administration. She has no palpable pulse, and the cardiac monitor shows ventricular fibrillation. The nurse immediately calls a code blue and begins chest compressions.

You are the charge nurse and designated code team leader for this shift. This is your responsibility to coordinate the resuscitation effort, make critical decisions about interventions, and ensure effective team communication during this emergency. The code team includes a respiratory therapist, pharmacist, resident physician, and several nurses with varying levels of experience (60).

Initial Assessment Upon Arrival: Mrs. Washington is unconscious and pulseless. The primary nurse is performing effective chest compressions. The cardiac monitor confirms ventricular fibrillation. IV access is patent from her previous admission. No obvious cause for the arrest is immediately apparent.

Team Member Assignments:

- **Primary nurse**: Continuing chest compressions (high quality)

- **Secondary nurse**: Preparing defibrillator and medications

- **Respiratory therapist**: Managing airway and ventilation

- **Resident physician**: Available for procedures and medication orders

- **Pharmacist**: Preparing and calculating emergency medications

- **You (Charge nurse)**: Code team leader and decision coordinator

NGN-Style Timed Decision Points:

Time 0 minutes - Code initiation: Immediate Actions (Select appropriate sequence): A. Verify pulselessness and rhythm B. Ensure high-quality CPR is in progress
C. Charge defibrillator to 200 joules D. Assign team member roles clearly E. Prepare emergency medications

Correct Sequence: A, B, D, C, E

Time 1 minute - First intervention cycle: High-quality CPR has been ongoing. Defibrillator is charged and ready.

Your Leadership Decision: "Stop compressions. Check rhythm. All clear for shock."

Post-shock Protocol (Select next actions): A. Immediately resume chest compressions for 2 minutes B. Check pulse and rhythm immediately after shock C. Administer epinephrine 1 mg IV push D. Continue ventilation with bag-mask device E. Prepare amiodarone for next rhythm check

Correct Actions: A, C, D, E (but NOT B)

Rationale: Current ACLS guidelines recommend immediate resumption of compressions after defibrillation without pulse check. Epinephrine should be given as soon as IV access is available. Amiodarone is prepared for refractory VF/VT (61).

Time 3 minutes - Second rhythm check: After 2 minutes of high-quality CPR and epinephrine administration, you call for rhythm check.

Rhythm Analysis: Monitor shows ventricular fibrillation persists.

Your Next Leadership Decision: "Still in VF. Continue compressions while I charge the defibrillator to 200 joules. Amiodarone ready?"

Second Shock Sequence:

1. Ensure all team members are clear

2. Deliver second defibrillation

3. Immediately resume compressions

4. Administer amiodarone 300 mg IV push

5. Continue 2-minute cycle

Time 5 minutes - Third rhythm check: **Monitor Assessment**: Rhythm has changed to normal sinus rhythm at rate 85 bpm.

Critical Decision Point: "Stop compressions. Check pulse."

Pulse Check Result: Strong carotid and radial pulses palpable, blood pressure 110/70.

Post-Resuscitation Care Priorities:

1. Maintain continuous cardiac monitoring

2. Assess neurological status and responsiveness

3. Obtain 12-lead EKG and chest X-ray

4. Transfer to intensive care unit for monitoring

5. Investigate underlying cause of arrest

Team Debriefing Session: After Mrs. Washington is stabilized and transferred to ICU, you conduct a brief team debriefing to review the resuscitation effort, identify what went well, and discuss areas for improvement. This educational opportunity helps team members learn from the experience and improve future code responses.

Scenario 44: Massive Transfusion Protocol

Patient Background: Sarah Martinez, a 35-year-old emergency department nurse, arrives as a trauma patient following a high-speed motor vehicle accident. She was the unrestrained driver of a vehicle that collided with a tree at approximately 45 mph. Initial assessment reveals multiple injuries including suspected internal bleeding, and the trauma team activates the massive transfusion protocol due to signs of hemorrhagic shock and hemodynamic instability.

Initial trauma assessment shows blunt abdominal trauma with likely liver laceration, multiple rib fractures, and significant blood loss. Her blood pressure is 70/40, heart rate 140, and she's showing signs of class III hemorrhagic shock. The blood bank has been notified to prepare emergency blood products, and the trauma surgeon is preparing for emergency surgical intervention (62).

Current Status: Sarah is intubated and mechanically ventilated, with two large-bore IV lines and central venous access for rapid volume resuscitation. Initial laboratory results show hemoglobin 6.2 g/dL, hematocrit 18%, platelets 145,000/μL, INR 1.8, and lactate 5.2 mmol/L indicating significant hemorrhagic shock.

Massive Transfusion Protocol Components:

- **Red blood cells**: 6 units O-negative (universal donor) immediately available

- **Fresh frozen plasma**: 6 units to correct coagulopathy

- **Platelets**: 1 apheresis unit to maintain hemostasis

- **Cryoprecipitate**: Available if fibrinogen levels drop below 100 mg/dL

NGN-Style Bowtie for Resuscitation Priorities:

Central Problem: 35-year-old trauma patient with hemorrhagic shock requiring massive transfusion

Assessment Parameters (Select all that apply):

- Hemoglobin and hematocrit trends

- Coagulation studies (PT/INR, aPTT)

- Platelet count and function

- Lactate levels for tissue perfusion

- Vital signs and hemodynamic status

- Signs of transfusion reactions

- Core body temperature

Transfusion Management (Select all that apply):

- Administer blood products in balanced ratios

- Monitor for signs of transfusion reactions

- Maintain patient normothermia

- Correct coagulopathy with plasma and platelets

- Use blood warmers for all products

- Document all blood product administration

- Coordinate with blood bank for ongoing supply

Monitoring and Support (Select all that apply):

- Continuous hemodynamic monitoring

- Serial laboratory assessments

- Watch for complications (TRALI, TACO, DIC)

- Electrolyte monitoring (especially calcium)

- Acid-base status assessment

- Surgical coordination for source control

Correct Selections: All listed items are appropriate for massive transfusion protocol management.

Balanced Resuscitation Strategy: The massive transfusion protocol follows a 1:1:1 ratio approach—for every unit of red blood cells, one unit of plasma and one unit of platelets (or equivalent) are administered. This balanced approach reduces mortality compared to older strategies that focused primarily on red blood cell replacement.

Hour 1 - Initial Resuscitation:

- 4 units packed red blood cells

- 4 units fresh frozen plasma

- 1 apheresis platelet unit

- Continuous monitoring for transfusion reactions

Laboratory Response After Initial Transfusion:

- **Hemoglobin**: 8.1 g/dL (improved)

- **INR**: 1.4 (improving)

- **Platelets**: 110,000/μL (adequate)

- **Lactate**: 4.1 mmol/L (improving)

- **Blood pressure**: 95/60 (stabilizing)

Ongoing Management: Sarah undergoes emergency surgery for liver repair and spleen removal. The surgical team achieves hemostasis, and she requires 2 additional units of red blood cells during the procedure. Her condition stabilizes, and she's transferred to the trauma ICU for ongoing monitoring and recovery.

Scenario 45: Disaster Response Triage

Patient Background: A multi-vehicle accident on a major highway during rush hour has resulted in 23 casualties arriving at your hospital within a 45-minute period. As the charge nurse in the emergency department, you must coordinate triage decisions, resource allocation, and patient flow while ensuring that the most critically injured patients receive immediate attention. The hospital's disaster response plan has been activated, but resources remain limited relative to the number and severity of injuries.

The accident involved a tour bus, three passenger vehicles, and a commercial truck carrying hazardous materials. Casualties range from minor injuries to life-threatening trauma, and several patients require immediate surgical intervention. The hospital's blood bank, operating rooms, and intensive care unit are all operating at capacity, requiring difficult decisions about resource prioritization (72).

Disaster Triage Categories: The START (Simple Triage and Rapid Treatment) system guides initial patient sorting based on severity of injury and likelihood of survival with available resources. Each patient receives a color-coded designation that determines treatment priority and resource allocation.

NGN-Style Matrix for Priority Setting:

Patient Presentation Analysis (Categorize each patient):

Patient A: 45-year-old unconscious with head trauma, dilated pupils, abnormal posturing

- **Respiratory status**: Agonal breathing pattern, requiring ventilatory support

- **Perfusion status**: Weak pulse, hypotensive

- **Neurological status**: Glasgow Coma Scale 3, poor prognosis

- **Triage category**: Red (immediate) vs. Black (expectant)

Patient B: 32-year-old alert and oriented with open femur fracture and stable vital signs

- **Respiratory status**: Normal, speaking in full sentences

- **Perfusion status**: Adequate, controlled bleeding

- **Neurological status**: Alert and oriented

- **Triage category**: Yellow (delayed)

Patient C: 28-year-old in respiratory distress with flail chest and pneumothorax

- **Respiratory status**: Severe distress, paradoxical chest movement

- **Perfusion status**: Tachycardic but adequate blood pressure

- **Neurological status**: Alert but anxious

- **Triage category**: Red (immediate)

Patient D: 55-year-old walking wounded with lacerations and minor burns

- **Respiratory status**: Normal

- **Perfusion status**: Stable vital signs

- **Neurological status**: Alert and oriented

- **Triage category**: Green (minor)

Triage Decision Framework:

Red (Immediate): Life-threatening injuries with high survival probability with immediate treatment. These patients receive immediate access to operating rooms, blood products, and intensive care resources.

Yellow (Delayed): Serious but not immediately life-threatening injuries. Treatment can be delayed 2-4 hours without significantly affecting survival. These patients are monitored closely for deterioration.

Green (Minor): Minor injuries that can be treated with basic first aid. These patients may be discharged home or transferred to minor treatment areas to free up emergency department space.

Black (Expectant): Injuries incompatible with survival given available resources, or requiring resources that would compromise care for other patients with better survival prospects.

Resource Allocation Challenges:

Operating Room Assignment: Three patients require emergency surgery, but only two operating rooms are available. Priority goes to patients with highest survival probability and greatest benefit from immediate intervention.

Blood Product Management: Multiple patients require blood transfusion, but blood bank supplies are limited. Type O-negative blood is reserved for most critical patients while type-specific blood is obtained for others.

ICU Bed Allocation: Five patients require intensive care monitoring, but only two ICU beds are available. Patients are prioritized based on severity of illness and need for specialized monitoring or interventions.

Scenario 46: Deteriorating Patient Recognition

Patient Background: Dorothy Chen, a 72-year-old retired librarian, was admitted 48 hours ago for routine cholecystectomy that was completed without complications. Her initial recovery progressed normally, and she was transferred to the medical-surgical unit yesterday evening. However, her day shift nurse noted subtle changes in her condition that don't fit typical post-operative patterns, raising concerns about early signs of clinical deterioration.

Mrs. Chen's changes are subtle but concerning: she seems less engaged in conversation, her appetite has decreased, she's complained of mild nausea, and her vital signs show trends that individually appear normal but collectively suggest early physiological compromise. These early warning signs require skilled nursing assessment and judgment to determine if intervention is needed (73).

Subtle Clinical Changes Assessment:

- **Mental status**: Less talkative than yesterday, takes longer to respond to questions

- **Appetite**: Refusing most meals, only taking small sips of water

- **Activity level**: Reluctant to ambulate, reports feeling "tired"

- **Vital sign trends**: Heart rate increased from 75 to 95, blood pressure slightly lower than baseline

- **Skin changes**: Slightly pale, skin feels cooler than previously noted

Early Warning Score Calculation: The Modified Early Warning Score (MEWS) helps quantify subtle changes that might indicate clinical deterioration. Each parameter is scored, and the total score guides intervention decisions.

NGN-Style Highlighting Critical Cues:

Review Mrs. Chen's assessment data and highlight findings that indicate need for immediate evaluation:

"Mrs. Chen is 48 hours post-operative from uncomplicated cholecystectomy. Today she appears less engaged in conversation and takes longer to respond to questions. Her appetite has decreased significantly, refusing most meals and taking only small sips of water. She reports feeling tired and is reluctant to ambulate as ordered. Her heart rate has increased from baseline 75 to 95 bpm, and blood pressure has decreased slightly from her normal range. Her skin appears paler than yesterday and feels cooler to touch. She reports mild nausea but denies pain at the surgical site."

Critical Cues to Highlight:

- appears less engaged in conversation and takes longer to respond to questions

- appetite has decreased significantly, refusing most meals

- heart rate has increased from baseline 75 to 95 bpm

- blood pressure has decreased slightly from her normal range

- skin appears paler than yesterday and feels cooler to touch

Rationale: These findings suggest early sepsis or other serious complications. Mental status changes, decreased oral intake, tachycardia, and perfusion changes require immediate evaluation. Early recognition and intervention can prevent progression to organ failure (74).

Early Intervention Protocol:

Immediate Assessment:

1. Complete vital signs including temperature and oxygen saturation

2. Focused physical examination including surgical site assessment

3. Laboratory studies including complete blood count, basic metabolic panel, lactate

4. Blood cultures if fever or elevated white blood cell count

5. Chest X-ray to rule out pneumonia or other pulmonary complications

Physician Notification: Using SBAR (Situation, Background, Assessment, Recommendation) format to communicate concerns clearly and request immediate evaluation.

Monitoring Enhancement: Increase vital sign frequency to every 2 hours and implement continuous pulse oximetry monitoring until patient stability is confirmed.

Advanced Clinical Leadership and Ethical Decision-Making

These advanced scenarios demonstrate the complexity of critical care nursing that extends beyond technical skills to include leadership abilities, resource management, and ethical reasoning. Each situation requires you to integrate clinical knowledge with professional judgment and communication expertise while coordinating care across multiple disciplines and stakeholders.

Crisis Leadership Skills: Managing multiple organ failure, coordinating disaster response, and recognizing subtle clinical deterioration all require leadership skills that develop through experience and deliberate practice. Your ability to remain calm under pressure, communicate clearly, and make difficult decisions directly impacts patient outcomes.

Resource Management: Advanced scenarios often involve limited resources requiring difficult allocation decisions. Understanding how to prioritize interventions, coordinate with other departments, and optimize available resources represents sophisticated nursing practice.

Ethical Reasoning: Complex medical situations frequently involve competing values, uncertain outcomes, and difficult family dynamics. Your role includes helping navigate these challenges while maintaining focus on patient-centered care and professional integrity.

Professional Excellence in Critical Situations

These scenarios prepare you for the most demanding aspects of nursing practice where clinical expertise, leadership skills, and ethical reasoning converge. The ability to manage complex medical emergencies, lead healthcare teams, and advocate for patients and families represents the highest level of nursing practice.

Each case builds upon previous knowledge while introducing new concepts about advanced pathophysiology, complex therapeutic interventions, and professional responsibilities. The integration of clinical expertise with leadership skills and ethical reasoning reflects the reality that advanced nursing practice extends far beyond bedside technical skills to include mentoring others, contributing to quality improvement, and serving as a clinical resource for complex patient situations.

Chapter 18: Complex Ethical and System Scenarios

Scenario 47: End-of-Life Care Decisions

Patient Background: Frank Wilson, an 85-year-old retired postal worker, has been in the medical ICU for three weeks with multi-organ failure following complications from pneumonia that progressed to septic shock. Despite aggressive treatment including mechanical ventilation, continuous renal replacement therapy, and multiple vasoactive medications, his condition continues to deteriorate. His family is struggling with decisions about continuing life-sustaining treatments.

Mr. Wilson's medical history includes diabetes, hypertension, mild dementia, and chronic kidney disease. Before this illness, he lived in an assisted living facility and required help with some activities of daily living but enjoyed visits from his children and grandchildren. He never completed advance directives, and his family reports that he never discussed his wishes for end-of-life care in detail (63).

Current Medical Status: Mr. Wilson requires maximum ventilator support, continuous dialysis, and three vasoactive medications to maintain blood pressure. His mental status shows no meaningful response to stimulation. Recent imaging suggests possible anoxic brain injury, and multiple organ systems are failing despite intensive support.

Family Dynamics: His three adult children have different perspectives on continuing treatment. His daughter (medical power of attorney) wants "everything possible" done, believing her father would want to "keep fighting." His two sons express concerns about prolonging suffering and question if continuing aggressive treatment aligns with their father's values and dignity.

Healthcare Team Assessment: The intensivist, primary nurse, chaplain, and social worker have met to discuss Mr. Wilson's prognosis and treatment options. The medical consensus is that recovery to meaningful function is extremely unlikely, and current treatments are sustaining biological life but not addressing the underlying disease process.

NGN-Style Multiple Perspectives Analysis:

Ethical Principles in Conflict:

Autonomy Considerations:

- Patient's previously expressed values and preferences (limited information available)

- Family's role as surrogate decision-makers

- Respecting patient's presumed wishes based on life history

Beneficence vs. Non-maleficence:

- Benefits of continuing life-sustaining treatment (preserving life)

- Harms of continuing treatment (prolonging suffering, preventing natural death)

- Quality vs. quantity of life considerations

Justice Considerations:

- Resource allocation and ICU bed availability

- Family's right to make decisions vs. medical team's assessment

- Societal expectations about end-of-life care

Family Meeting Facilitation:

Meeting Participants:

- Mr. Wilson's three children and two grandchildren

- Attending physician (intensivist)

- Primary nurse

- Hospital chaplain
- Social worker

Meeting Objectives:

1. Provide clear, honest information about Mr. Wilson's condition and prognosis

2. Explore the family's understanding of the situation

3. Discuss treatment options including comfort care

4. Support family decision-making process

5. Address emotional and spiritual needs

Communication Strategies:

- Use clear, non-medical language to explain condition
- Allow time for questions and emotional responses
- Avoid pressuring family toward specific decisions
- Focus on what Mr. Wilson would have wanted
- Provide information about palliative and hospice care options

Case Resolution: After extensive family discussions and consultation with the palliative care team, the family decides to transition to comfort care measures. Life-sustaining treatments are gradually withdrawn, and Mr. Wilson is transferred to the palliative care unit where he dies peacefully with his family present three days later.

Professional Leadership and Ethical Reasoning

These advanced scenarios demonstrate the complexity of critical care nursing that extends beyond technical skills to include leadership abilities, ethical reasoning, and communication expertise. Each situation requires you to integrate clinical knowledge with professional judgment and interpersonal skills.

Leadership Development: Code blue leadership requires clear communication, decisive action, and the ability to coordinate multiple team members under extreme pressure. These skills transfer to other emergency situations and everyday charge nurse responsibilities.

Ethical Decision-Making: End-of-life scenarios challenge you to balance competing ethical principles while supporting families through difficult decisions. Understanding your role in ethical deliberation and family advocacy represents advanced nursing practice.

Crisis Management: Massive transfusion protocols and cardiogenic shock management require systematic approaches to complex medical emergencies while maintaining attention to patient safety and family needs.

Professional Growth Opportunities

These scenarios prepare you for leadership roles in critical care settings where you'll be expected to make complex decisions, coordinate care across multiple disciplines, and provide guidance to less experienced nurses. The integration of clinical expertise with leadership skills and ethical reasoning represents the highest level of nursing practice.

Each case builds upon previous knowledge while introducing new concepts about advanced pathophysiology, complex therapeutic interventions, and professional responsibilities. The emphasis on interdisciplinary collaboration, family communication, and ethical reasoning reflects the reality that advanced nursing practice extends far beyond bedside technical skills.

Contemplations on Advanced Practice

Advanced critical care scenarios remind us that nursing at its highest level involves not just managing complex medical conditions, but leading healthcare teams, advocating for patients and families, and making difficult ethical decisions under pressure. Your role as an advanced practitioner includes mentoring others, contributing to quality improvement initiatives, and serving as a clinical resource for complex patient situations.

The scenarios in this section prepare you for the most challenging aspects of nursing practice while emphasizing the importance of maintaining compassion, professional integrity, and commitment to patient-centered care even in the most difficult circumstances.

Key Learning Points

- Cardiogenic shock requires sophisticated hemodynamic monitoring and mechanical circulatory support

- Code blue leadership demands clear communication, decisive action, and effective team coordination

- Massive transfusion protocols follow balanced resuscitation strategies with continuous monitoring for complications

- End-of-life care decisions require ethical reasoning, family communication, and interdisciplinary collaboration

- Advanced practice nursing integrates clinical expertise with leadership skills and ethical reasoning

- Crisis management requires systematic approaches while maintaining attention to patient safety and family needs

- Professional leadership includes mentoring others and contributing to quality improvement initiatives

- Ethical decision-making involves balancing competing principles while advocating for patient and family needs

- Communication skills become increasingly important as clinical situations become more complex

- Advanced nursing practice extends beyond technical skills to include professional judgment and moral reasoning

Scenario 48: Capacity and Consent Issues

Patient Background: Dorothy Chen, a 78-year-old retired librarian with mild cognitive impairment, presents to the emergency department with signs of stroke requiring urgent intervention. She arrived alone after neighbors found her confused and unable to speak clearly. The stroke team recommends tissue plasminogen activator (tPA) treatment, but Mrs. Chen appears to refuse consent, shaking her head and pushing away medical staff when they approach with consent forms.

Mrs. Chen lives alone in her apartment and has been managing independently despite gradually worsening memory problems over the past two years. Her primary care physician has noted mild cognitive impairment but she's maintained decision-making capacity for routine medical decisions. However, her current neurological impairment from the stroke complicates assessment of her ability to understand and consent to emergency treatment (86).

Clinical Presentation: Mrs. Chen presents with sudden onset of right-sided weakness, facial droop, and severe expressive aphasia. Her NIHSS (National Institutes of Health Stroke Scale) score is 18, indicating severe stroke. CT angiogram shows large vessel occlusion in the left middle cerebral artery territory. She's within the time window for both IV tPA and mechanical thrombectomy, which could significantly improve her outcomes.

Capacity Assessment Challenges: Mrs. Chen's stroke affects her language centers, making traditional capacity assessment difficult. She appears alert and follows some simple commands, but cannot verbally communicate her understanding of proposed treatments or their risks and benefits. Her behavior suggests possible refusal of treatment, but determining if this represents informed decision-making or confusion from her stroke proves challenging.

Emergency Decision-Making Framework: The situation requires balancing respect for patient autonomy with the potential benefits of time-sensitive treatment. The emergency team must determine Mrs. Chen's decision-making capacity while considering legal and ethical frameworks for emergency treatment of patients with impaired capacity.

NGN-Style Decision Tree Navigation:

Initial Assessment Branch: Does Mrs. Chen have capacity to make treatment decisions?

Capacity Evaluation Criteria:

1. **Understanding:** Can she understand the nature of her condition and proposed treatment?

2. **Appreciation:** Does she appreciate how the information applies to her situation?

3. **Reasoning:** Can she manipulate information rationally to reach a decision?

4. **Choice communication:** Can she communicate a stable choice?

Assessment Results:

*   **Understanding:** Limited by aphasia, unclear if she grasps stroke severity

*   **Appreciation:** Cannot assess due to communication barriers

*   **Reasoning:** No evidence of rational decision-making process

*   **Choice communication:** Appears to refuse but unable to explain reasoning

Decision Tree Pathway A - Patient Has Capacity: If capacity is present, respect her apparent refusal and provide supportive care only, even if this leads to worse outcomes.

Decision Tree Pathway B - Patient Lacks Capacity: If capacity is absent, consider emergency treatment based on presumed consent doctrine, best interests, or surrogate decision-maker input.

Assessment Conclusion: Given the severity of her stroke, communication barriers, and inability to demonstrate understanding of consequences, the team determines Mrs. Chen currently lacks capacity for this specific decision.

Emergency Treatment Authorization: Under the emergency doctrine and presumed consent principles, the team proceeds with IV tPA administration while simultaneously attempting to contact family members or friends who might provide insight into her values and preferences.

Healthcare-Associated Complications and System Analysis

Scenario 49: Healthcare-Associated Complications

Patient Background: Robert Martinez, a 60-year-old maintenance supervisor, develops two serious healthcare-associated complications during what should have been a routine hospitalization for diabetic foot infection treatment. He acquires both a central line-associated bloodstream infection (CLABSI) and Clostridioides difficile colitis during his three-week stay, raising questions about infection control practices and system-level patient safety issues.

Mr. Martinez was admitted for IV antibiotic treatment of a diabetic foot ulcer that had not responded to outpatient oral antibiotics. His initial treatment plan involved 10-14 days of IV vancomycin and piperacillin-tazobactam through a peripherally inserted central catheter (PICC line). However, complications have extended his stay significantly and raised concerns about preventable harm (87).

Timeline of Complications:

Day 1-7: Routine care with PICC line insertion and IV antibiotic therapy. Patient progressing well with improving foot infection and stable blood glucose control.

Day 8: Patient develops fever and elevated white blood cell count. Blood cultures drawn from PICC line and peripheral sites grow methicillin-resistant Staphylococcus epidermidis, confirming CLABSI.

Day 12: After starting broad-spectrum antibiotics for CLABSI treatment, patient develops severe diarrhea. C. difficile toxin test returns positive, confirming healthcare-associated C. difficile infection.

Day 15-21: Patient requires isolation precautions, additional antibiotics, and extended hospitalization for treatment of both complications.

NGN-Style Root Cause Analysis:

CLABSI Investigation Factors:

Line Insertion Practices:

- **Sterile technique**: Review of procedure notes indicates proper sterile technique documented

- **Site selection**: PICC placed in appropriate location without complications

- **Operator experience**: Placed by experienced vascular access team member

Line Maintenance Issues:

- **Daily necessity assessment**: Chart review shows line necessity assessed daily initially, then missed for 3 days

- **Dressing changes**: Some delays in scheduled dressing changes due to staffing issues

- **Hub disinfection**: Inconsistent documentation of hub scrubbing before access

Environmental Factors:

- **Hand hygiene compliance**: Unit compliance rate 78% (below 90% target)

- **Staff workload**: Higher than normal patient-to-nurse ratios during middle weekend

- **Equipment availability**: Temporary shortage of chlorhexidine dressing supplies

C. Difficile Analysis Factors:

Antibiotic Stewardship:

- **Initial therapy**: Appropriate narrow-spectrum choice for foot infection

- **CLABSI treatment**: Broad-spectrum therapy necessary but prolonged duration

- **PPI use**: Patient on omeprazole, which increases C. diff risk

Infection Control Practices:

- **Hand hygiene**: Same compliance issues noted for CLABSI

- **Environmental cleaning**: Terminal cleaning protocols followed but daily cleaning inconsistent

- **Isolation practices**: Some delays in implementing contact precautions for other C. diff patients

System-Level Contributing Factors:

- **Staffing patterns**: Weekend and evening shift understaffing

- **Education gaps**: Some staff unfamiliar with updated CLABSI prevention protocols

- **Communication issues**: Inconsistent shift handoff about line care requirements

Quality Improvement Response: The hospital's infection control team initiates targeted interventions addressing identified system issues including enhanced staff education, improved hand hygiene monitoring, standardized line care protocols, and environmental cleaning audits.

Complex Discharge Planning

Scenario 50: Complex Discharge Planning

Patient Background: Margaret Washington, a 75-year-old retired teacher, requires complex discharge planning following hospitalization for heart failure exacerbation complicated by acute kidney injury, medication-induced delirium, and new mobility limitations. She has multiple chronic conditions requiring ongoing management and lives alone in a two-story home that may no longer be safe for independent living.

Mrs. Washington's hospitalization began with routine heart failure management but became complicated when her home medications (including high-dose diuretics and NSAIDs for arthritis) contributed to acute kidney injury. Medication adjustments and new prescriptions led to confusion and agitation, requiring psychiatric consultation and medication changes. Prolonged bed rest resulted in significant functional decline, raising questions about her ability to return home safely (88).

Discharge Planning Challenges:

Medical Complexity:

- **Multiple conditions**: Heart failure, chronic kidney disease, diabetes, osteoarthritis, mild cognitive impairment

- **Medication changes**: Seven medication adjustments during hospitalization requiring education and monitoring

- **Follow-up needs**: Cardiology, nephrology, primary care, and physical therapy appointments scheduled

Functional Assessment:

- **Mobility decline**: Requires walker for ambulation, unable to climb stairs safely

- **Cognitive status**: Mild baseline impairment worsened by hospital delirium, now improving but not back to baseline

- **Activities of daily living**: Needs assistance with bathing, medication management, and meal preparation

Social and Environmental Factors:

- **Living situation**: Lives alone in two-story home, bedroom and bathroom upstairs

- **Family support**: Daughter lives 200 miles away, visits monthly but unable to provide daily assistance

- **Financial resources**: Limited income, Medicare coverage with gaps in home care benefits

NGN-Style Comprehensive Discharge Checklist:

Medical Management Coordination:

- **Medication reconciliation**: Complete review of all medications with clear instructions and pill organizer setup

- **Laboratory monitoring**: Scheduled for kidney function and electrolyte monitoring within 48 hours of discharge

- **Follow-up appointments**: Cardiology in 1 week, primary care in 3 days, nephrology in 2 weeks

- **Emergency planning**: Clear instructions about when to seek immediate medical attention

Safety Assessment and Modifications:

- **Home safety evaluation**: Occupational therapy assessment identifies needed modifications

- **Fall prevention**: Remove scatter rugs, install grab bars, improve lighting

- **Medical alert system**: Arrange for emergency response system given living alone

- **Medication safety**: Pill organizer setup with pharmacy consultation for delivery services

Support Services Coordination:

- **Home health nursing**: Three visits per week for medication monitoring and symptom assessment

- **Physical therapy**: Home-based therapy to address mobility and strength deficits

- **Meal delivery**: Arrange for healthy meal delivery service for cardiac and diabetic diet

- **Transportation**: Medical transport for follow-up appointments given inability to drive

Communication and Education:

- **Patient education**: Written instructions in large print about medications, diet, symptoms to report

- **Family involvement**: Daughter included in all discharge education via phone conference

- **Primary care communication**: Detailed discharge summary sent to all providers

- **Emergency information**: Wallet card with current medications and emergency contacts

Case Resolution: Mrs. Washington is discharged to her home with extensive support services. Home modifications are completed before discharge, and she demonstrates understanding of her medications and when to seek help. Follow-up at one week shows successful transition with stable vital signs and no major complications.

Ethical Leadership in Complex Healthcare Systems

These advanced scenarios demonstrate how nursing practice intersects with broader ethical, legal, and system-level considerations that shape healthcare delivery. Each situation requires integration of clinical knowledge with ethical reasoning, communication skills, and system-level thinking to optimize patient outcomes while maintaining professional integrity.

Ethical Decision-Making Skills: End-of-life care scenarios require balancing respect for autonomy with beneficence and non-maleficence while supporting families through difficult decisions. Capacity assessment involves applying legal and ethical frameworks to protect patient rights while ensuring appropriate care.

System-Level Analysis: Healthcare-associated complications require understanding of how individual practices connect to system-level outcomes, quality improvement methodologies, and root cause analysis techniques to prevent future harm.

Care Coordination Excellence: Complex discharge planning demands sophisticated understanding of healthcare systems, community resources, and interdisciplinary collaboration to ensure successful transitions and prevent readmissions.

Professional Growth Through Ethical Practice

These scenarios prepare you for leadership roles where you'll face complex ethical decisions, participate in quality improvement initiatives, and coordinate care for patients with multiple needs across various healthcare settings. The integration of clinical expertise with ethical reasoning and system-level thinking represents the highest level of nursing practice.

Each case builds upon previous knowledge while introducing concepts about healthcare ethics, quality improvement, care coordination, and professional responsibilities. The emphasis on patient advocacy, family communication, and system-level improvement reflects the reality that advanced nursing practice extends far beyond individual patient care to include broader professional and social responsibilities.

Continuing the Journey

These final scenarios remind us that nursing practice exists within complex healthcare systems where individual decisions have broader implications for patients, families, and communities. Your role as a professional nurse includes not just providing excellent bedside care but also advocating for patients, supporting families, improving systems, and maintaining ethical standards that honor the profession's commitment to human welfare.

The knowledge and skills you develop through engaging with these scenarios will serve you throughout your nursing career as you encounter new challenges, advance in leadership roles, and contribute to the ongoing development of nursing practice. The ethical foundations and system-level thinking you develop now will guide your decision-making and professional growth for years to come.

Each scenario in this book has prepared you for different aspects of nursing practice, from basic clinical skills to advanced ethical reasoning. Together, they provide a foundation for lifelong learning, professional development, and service to others that defines the essence of professional nursing practice.

Key Learning Points

- End-of-life care decisions require balancing multiple ethical principles while supporting family consensus-building

- Capacity assessment for emergency treatment involves applying legal and ethical frameworks under time pressure

- Healthcare-associated complications demand system-level analysis and quality improvement responses

- Complex discharge planning requires coordination across multiple disciplines and community resources

- Ethical leadership integrates clinical expertise with broader professional and social responsibilities

- Family communication during difficult decisions requires structured approaches and emotional support

- Root cause analysis identifies system-level factors contributing to preventable patient harm

- Interdisciplinary collaboration becomes increasingly important as patient complexity increases

- Professional nursing practice extends beyond bedside care to include advocacy and system improvement

- Continuous learning and ethical reflection are essential for advanced nursing practice

Chapter 19: Integrating Scenarios into Clinical Practice

The gap between classroom learning and clinical reality often surprises nursing students. You might excel at answering questions about patient scenarios in controlled academic settings, yet feel overwhelmed when facing similar situations with real patients who don't follow textbook presentations exactly. This chapter addresses how to bridge that gap effectively, transforming scenario-based learning into confident clinical practice.

Bridging Classroom to Clinical

The transition from theoretical knowledge to practical application represents one of the most challenging aspects of nursing education. Scenarios provide a crucial bridge in this process, offering structured practice opportunities that mirror clinical decision-making without the pressure and unpredictability of real patient care.

Pre-Clinical Preparation Strategies

Effective preparation for clinical experiences involves more than reviewing pathophysiology and nursing procedures. You need to develop systematic approaches to patient assessment, clinical reasoning, and decision-making that you can apply consistently across different patient situations.

Mental rehearsal using scenarios helps you practice clinical reasoning processes before encountering similar situations in practice. Work through scenarios that relate to your upcoming clinical area, focusing not just on correct answers but on developing systematic approaches to patient assessment and care planning.

Consider this approach: Before your medical-surgical rotation, work through scenarios involving common conditions you're likely to encounter—heart failure, COPD exacerbations, post-operative care, diabetes management. Pay attention to the assessment patterns, intervention priorities, and monitoring requirements that appear consistently across similar patients.

Conceptual preparation involves understanding the underlying principles that guide nursing care rather than memorizing specific procedures or protocols. When you understand why certain interventions are used and how they relate to patient pathophysiology, you can adapt your approach when situations don't match exactly what you've studied.

For example, rather than memorizing that heart failure patients need daily weights, understand that fluid retention is a key indicator of disease progression and that weight changes provide early warning of decompensation. This understanding allows you to apply the principle to different patients with varying presentations and comorbidities.

Skill integration practice helps you connect clinical reasoning with psychomotor skills. Scenarios help you think through when and why you might use specific skills, not just how to perform them. This integration is crucial because clinical practice requires simultaneous attention to cognitive and technical aspects of care.

Case Example: Pre-Clinical Integration

Sarah is preparing for her first medical-surgical clinical rotation. She works through Scenario 4 (Basic Heart Failure Management) and focuses on understanding the clinical reasoning process:

She identifies that Mrs. Washington's weight gain pattern (5 pounds in 5 days) indicates fluid retention, not just random weight fluctuation. She connects this finding to the pathophysiology of heart failure—decreased cardiac output leads to fluid retention, which worsens cardiac workload and can precipitate acute decompensation.

When Sarah encounters a similar patient in clinical practice, she doesn't just follow orders to weigh the patient daily. She understands what the weights mean, anticipates what changes might indicate, and can communicate meaningfully with the healthcare team about the patient's status. This deeper understanding enables more sophisticated clinical reasoning and better patient advocacy.

Post-Clinical Reflection Using Scenarios

Post-clinical reflection transforms clinical experiences into learning opportunities that accelerate professional development. However, unstructured reflection often lacks the depth needed for significant learning. Scenarios provide frameworks for systematic reflection that help you extract maximum learning from each clinical encounter.

Comparative analysis involves comparing your actual clinical experiences with similar scenarios, identifying what was similar, what was different, and what you might do differently in future situations. This analysis helps you recognize patterns in your clinical reasoning and identify areas for improvement.

After caring for a patient with pneumonia, for example, you might compare your experience with Scenario 7 (Community-Acquired Pneumonia). Did you recognize the same assessment priorities? How did your patient's presentation differ from the scenario? What interventions were most effective? What would you do differently next time?

Hypothesis testing uses scenarios to explore alternative approaches to clinical situations you've encountered. If you faced a challenging patient situation, work through similar scenarios to consider different assessment approaches, intervention options, or communication strategies you might have used.

Learning consolidation involves connecting clinical experiences with theoretical knowledge through scenario analysis. This process helps you understand not just what happened during patient care, but why certain approaches were effective and how you might apply similar reasoning to future situations.

Case Example: Post-Clinical Reflection

Mark cared for Mr. Rodriguez, a 58-year-old patient who developed chest pain during his shift. Mark followed protocols appropriately, obtaining an EKG and notifying the physician, but he felt uncertain about his assessment and worried he might have missed something important.

Using Scenario 21 (Acute Myocardial Infarction) for reflection, Mark analyzes his clinical reasoning process. He realizes he focused primarily on the chest pain itself but didn't systematically assess other indicators of cardiac problems—skin color, diaphoresis, nausea, or anxiety level. The scenario helps him understand how these additional cues might have provided important information about the severity and nature of Mr. Rodriguez's condition.

This reflection doesn't criticize Mark's care—his interventions were appropriate and effective. Instead, it helps him develop more sophisticated assessment skills for future similar situations. The scenario provides a framework for understanding expert clinical reasoning that he can apply to enhance his own practice.

Connecting Scenarios to Real Patients

Real patients rarely present exactly like textbook scenarios, but the clinical reasoning processes you practice with scenarios translate directly to patient care when you focus on underlying principles rather than surface details.

Pattern recognition transfer involves applying the assessment and reasoning patterns you learn from scenarios to patients with similar underlying problems, even when presentations vary. A patient with heart failure might not have exactly the same symptoms as Mrs. Washington in Scenario 4, but the principle of monitoring for fluid retention indicators remains constant.

Adaptability development comes from understanding why certain interventions are used, not just when to use them. This understanding allows you to modify your approach when patient circumstances don't match scenario parameters exactly.

Clinical grasp enhancement occurs when you practice identifying the most significant aspects of complex patient presentations. Scenarios help you develop this skill by highlighting which patient cues are most important and why they take priority over other available information.

Case Example: Pattern Recognition Transfer

Jessica learned from Scenario 6 (COPD Stable Management) that patients with COPD need careful assessment of respiratory status changes and patient education about medication use. When she encounters Mr. Peterson in clinical practice, his presentation differs somewhat from the scenario—he's having more difficulty with activities of daily living and seems more anxious about his condition.

Jessica applies the same clinical reasoning process she practiced with the scenario: she assesses his respiratory status systematically, evaluates his medication knowledge and technique, and explores what specific concerns are causing his anxiety. While his presentation differs from the scenario, the underlying assessment priorities and intervention principles remain the same.

Her scenario-based preparation allows her to focus on Mr. Peterson's individual needs rather than trying to remember specific protocols. This patient-centered approach leads to more effective care and greater confidence in her clinical judgment.

Building Clinical Confidence

Confidence in clinical practice develops gradually through successful experiences that build on one another. Scenarios provide controlled opportunities to practice clinical reasoning and experience success before encountering similar situations in higher-stakes clinical environments.

Systematic approach development helps build confidence by providing reliable frameworks for patient assessment and care planning. When you have systematic approaches to common clinical situations, you feel more prepared to handle unexpected variations or complications.

Decision-making practice through scenarios helps you develop comfort with the uncertainty inherent in clinical practice. Every patient situation involves some degree of ambiguity, and confidence comes from learning to make sound decisions despite incomplete information.

Success experience accumulation occurs when you consistently work through scenarios successfully and see improvement in your clinical reasoning abilities. This sense of growing competence transfers to clinical practice and supports confidence development.

Using Scenarios for NCLEX Preparation

While scenarios serve broader educational purposes, they also provide excellent preparation for the Next Generation NCLEX examination. However, effective NGN preparation involves more than just practicing question formats—it requires developing the clinical judgment skills that the examination is designed to assess.

Study Strategies for NGN Success

Systematic reasoning development represents the most important preparation strategy for NGN success. The examination assesses your ability to think through patient situations systematically, not your ability to recall specific facts or procedures. Focus your study efforts on developing consistent approaches to clinical reasoning that you can apply across different patient scenarios.

Use the Clinical Judgment Measurement Model as a framework for approaching each scenario: What cues do you recognize as significant? How do you analyze their meaning? What hypotheses do you prioritize? What solutions do you generate? How do you plan to implement interventions? How will you evaluate effectiveness?

This systematic approach serves you well not just on examinations, but throughout your nursing career. Developing these reasoning habits early in your education provides a foundation for lifelong professional growth.

Integration practice involves working with scenarios that combine multiple concepts or require you to apply knowledge from different content areas simultaneously. Real nursing practice rarely involves isolated problems, and the NGN reflects this reality by presenting complex scenarios that require integrated thinking.

Rather than studying cardiac conditions separately from diabetes management, for example, work through scenarios involving patients with both conditions. This approach helps you develop the kind of integrated thinking required for both examination success and clinical practice.

Time management skill development involves learning to work through complex scenarios efficiently without sacrificing thoroughness. The NGN allows more time per question than traditional formats, but scenarios are also more complex and require more sophisticated analysis.

Practice working through scenarios with attention to both accuracy and efficiency. Develop systematic approaches that help you identify relevant information quickly while ensuring you don't miss important cues or considerations.

Case Example: Integrated NGN Preparation

Amanda is preparing for the NGN and works through Scenario 28 (Diabetic Ketoacidosis). Rather than focusing only on getting questions correct, she practices systematic clinical reasoning:

She identifies relevant cues (blood glucose, pH, ketones, clinical symptoms), analyzes their significance (severe metabolic derangement requiring immediate intervention), prioritizes hypotheses (DKA with potential for life-threatening complications), generates solutions (fluid replacement, insulin therapy, electrolyte monitoring), plans implementation (IV access, continuous monitoring, frequent reassessment), and considers evaluation criteria (improving lab values, symptom resolution, stable vital signs).

This systematic approach prepares Amanda not just for examination questions about DKA, but for actually caring for patients with this condition. The clinical reasoning skills she develops through scenario practice serve her well in both examination and clinical contexts.

Creating Personal Scenario Banks

Developing your own collection of scenarios based on your clinical experiences helps personalize your learning and creates valuable study resources for future reference. Personal scenario banks allow you to focus on areas where you need additional practice and help you remember important clinical experiences more effectively.

Experience documentation involves creating written scenarios based on patients you've cared for, focusing on the clinical reasoning challenges they presented. This process helps consolidate learning from clinical experiences and creates resources for future study.

Pattern identification occurs when you analyze your personal scenarios to identify recurring themes, common challenges, or areas where you consistently struggle. This analysis helps you focus your study efforts on areas where additional practice would be most beneficial.

Peer collaboration through scenario sharing allows you to learn from your classmates' experiences while contributing your own insights to their learning. Different students encounter different types of patients, and sharing scenarios broadens everyone's exposure to varied clinical situations.

Peer Study Groups

Collaborative learning through peer study groups enhances scenario-based preparation by providing diverse perspectives on clinical reasoning and decision-making. Different students bring varied experiences, knowledge bases, and thinking styles that enrich everyone's learning.

Structured discussions using scenarios as focal points help ensure that study group time is productive and educational. Rather than simply comparing answers, discuss the reasoning processes that led to different conclusions and explore alternative approaches to patient care.

Role-playing exercises using scenarios help you practice clinical communication skills and experience patient situations from different perspectives. Taking turns playing the roles of nurse, patient, family member, or physician helps you understand the complexity of healthcare team dynamics.

Peer teaching opportunities through scenario explanations help solidify your own understanding while contributing to your peers' learning. Teaching others requires you to articulate your reasoning clearly and consider alternative perspectives, both valuable skills for clinical practice.

Self-Assessment Techniques

Regular self-assessment using scenarios helps you monitor your progress and identify areas needing additional focus. Effective self-assessment requires honest evaluation of your abilities and systematic tracking of your development over time.

Progress tracking involves maintaining records of your performance with different types of scenarios, noting areas of consistent strength and persistent challenges. This tracking helps you focus your study efforts efficiently and provides motivation as you see improvement over time.

Error analysis helps you understand not just when you make mistakes, but why those mistakes occur and how to prevent them in future situations. Look for patterns in your errors—do you consistently miss certain types of cues? Do you struggle with prioritization in specific types of situations?

Metacognitive reflection involves thinking about your thinking processes, analyzing how you approach clinical reasoning, and identifying strategies that work best for your learning style. This self-awareness accelerates learning and helps you develop more effective study strategies.

Lifelong Learning Applications

The clinical reasoning skills you develop through scenario-based learning serve you throughout your nursing career, not just during your initial education. Understanding how to apply these skills to ongoing professional development helps you maintain competence and continue growing as a professional.

Continuing Education Integration

Specialty preparation using scenarios relevant to your area of practice helps you develop expertise in specific clinical areas. Whether you're moving to critical care, pediatrics, or community health, scenario-based learning helps you develop the specialized clinical reasoning skills needed for different practice environments.

Competency maintenance through regular scenario practice helps you stay current with best practices and maintain sharp clinical reasoning skills. Just as athletes maintain their skills through regular practice, nurses can maintain clinical judgment abilities through ongoing scenario-based learning.

Evidence-based practice integration involves using scenarios to explore how new research findings might change your approach to patient care. When new evidence emerges about best practices for specific conditions, scenarios help you practice integrating this knowledge into your clinical reasoning.

Specialty Certification Preparation

Many nursing specialty certifications include clinical scenario components that assess your ability to apply specialized knowledge to patient care situations. The clinical reasoning skills you develop through general scenario practice provide a foundation for this specialized preparation.

Content-specific preparation involves working through scenarios that focus on your specialty area, paying attention to the unique assessment priorities, intervention strategies, and outcome evaluation methods relevant to your practice area.

Advanced reasoning development often requires more sophisticated clinical judgment skills than basic nursing practice. Specialty scenarios help you develop the advanced reasoning abilities needed for expert practice in specialized areas.

Preceptor Development

Experienced nurses who serve as preceptors for students or new graduates can use scenarios as teaching tools to help others develop clinical judgment skills. Understanding how to use scenarios effectively for teaching enhances your ability to contribute to the professional development of others.

Teaching skill development involves learning how to guide others through clinical reasoning processes rather than simply providing answers. Scenarios provide structured opportunities to practice these teaching skills in low-risk environments.

Assessment abilities for evaluating others' clinical reasoning development can be enhanced through your own scenario-based learning experiences. Understanding what constitutes effective clinical reasoning helps you evaluate and provide feedback to those you mentor.

Quality Improvement Projects

Healthcare organizations increasingly involve direct care nurses in quality improvement initiatives that require systematic analysis of patient care problems and development of evidence-based solutions. The analytical thinking skills you develop through scenario-based learning contribute to these broader professional responsibilities.

Systems thinking development involves understanding how individual patient care decisions fit into broader organizational and healthcare system contexts. Advanced scenarios that include system-level considerations help develop these important skills.

Data analysis skills for quality improvement often involve analyzing patterns in patient outcomes and identifying opportunities for improvement. The pattern recognition skills you develop through scenario analysis contribute to these analytical abilities.

Professional Growth and Leadership

As you advance in your nursing career, the clinical reasoning skills you develop through scenario-based learning provide a foundation for leadership roles, education responsibilities, and advanced practice opportunities.

Clinical expertise recognition often comes from your ability to think through complex patient situations and guide others in their clinical reasoning development. The systematic approaches you learn through scenario practice help you articulate your reasoning to others and serve as a clinical resource.

Mentorship capabilities develop as you become able to help others work through clinical reasoning challenges. Your experience with systematic clinical judgment development through scenarios prepares you to guide others through similar learning processes.

Moving Forward with Purpose

The scenarios in this book represent just the beginning of your clinical judgment development journey. The reasoning skills you practice here will evolve and deepen throughout your nursing career as you encounter new situations, gain experience, and continue learning.

The key to maximizing the value of scenario-based learning lies in approaching each scenario as an opportunity to develop systematic clinical reasoning skills rather than simply practicing for examinations. Focus on understanding the thinking processes that lead to sound clinical judgment, and you'll develop skills that serve you well in any clinical situation you encounter.

Clinical judgment represents both an art and a science—it requires both technical knowledge and the wisdom that comes from experience and reflection. Scenarios provide structured opportunities to develop both aspects of clinical reasoning in ways that prepare you for the complex realities of nursing practice.

Reflective Summary

The integration of scenario-based learning into clinical practice represents more than just an educational strategy—it provides a bridge between the theoretical knowledge you learn in classrooms and the complex realities you face in patient care. This bridge-building process requires intentional effort and systematic approaches, but the investment pays dividends throughout your nursing career.

The clinical reasoning abilities you develop through scenario practice become the foundation for confident, competent nursing practice. They enable you to approach patient care systematically, adapt to unexpected situations, and continue learning from each clinical encounter. Most importantly, they help you provide the kind of thoughtful, evidence-based care that represents the essence of professional nursing practice.

Key Learning Points

- Scenarios provide crucial bridges between theoretical knowledge and clinical practice application

- Pre-clinical preparation should focus on systematic clinical reasoning development rather than memorization

- Post-clinical reflection using scenarios helps extract maximum learning from clinical experiences

- Real patients rarely match scenarios exactly, but underlying clinical reasoning principles remain constant

- Confidence develops through systematic approaches and successful experiences that build on one another

- NGN preparation requires developing clinical judgment skills rather than just practicing question formats

- Personal scenario banks based on clinical experiences create valuable individualized learning resources

- Peer collaboration enhances learning through diverse perspectives and shared experiences

- Self-assessment techniques help monitor progress and identify areas needing additional focus

- Scenario-based reasoning skills serve lifelong learning and professional development needs

- Integration of scenarios into clinical practice requires intentional effort and systematic approaches

- Clinical judgment development represents both art and science requiring knowledge and experiential wisdom

Reference

1. Kavanagh, J. M., & Szweda, C. (2017). A crisis in competency: The strategic and ethical imperative to assessing new graduate nurses' clinical reasoning. *Nursing Education Perspectives*, 38(2), 57-62.

2. Duchscher, J. E. (2009). Transition shock: The initial stage of role adaptation for newly graduated registered nurses. *Journal of Advanced Nursing*, 65(5), 1103-1113.

3. Benner, P., Sutphen, M., Leonard, V., & Day, L. (2010). *Educating nurses: A call for radical transformation*. Jossey-Bass.

4. Kuiper, R., Pesut, D., & Kautz, D. (2009). Promoting the self-regulation of clinical reasoning skills in nursing students. *The Open Nursing Journal*, 3, 76-85.

5. Tanner, C. A. (2006). Thinking like a nurse: A research-based model of clinical judgment in nursing. *Journal of Nursing Education*, 45(6), 204-211.

6. Benner, P., & Tanner, C. (1987). Clinical judgment: How expert nurses use intuition. *American Journal of Nursing*, 87(1), 23-31.

7. Croskerry, P. (2009). A universal model of diagnostic reasoning. *Academic Medicine*, 84(8), 1022-1028.

8. Ericsson, K. A. (2008). Deliberate practice and acquisition of expert performance: A general overview. *Academic Emergency Medicine*, 15(11), 988-994.

9. Benner, P. (1984). *From novice to expert: Excellence and power in clinical nursing practice*. Addison-Wesley.

10. Lasater, K. (2007). Clinical judgment development: Using simulation to create an assessment rubric. *Journal of Nursing Education*, 46(11), 496-503.

11. Johns, C. (2013). *Becoming a reflective practitioner* (4th ed.). Wiley-Blackwell.

12. Tanner, C. A. (2006). Thinking like a nurse: A research-based model of clinical judgment in nursing. *Journal of Nursing Education*, 45(6), 204-211.

13. Lanas, A., & Chan, F. K. (2017). Peptic ulcer disease. *The Lancet*, 390(10094), 613-624.

14. Chey, W. D., Leontiadis, G. I., Howden, C. W., & Moss, S. F. (2017). ACG clinical guideline: Treatment of *Helicobacter pylori* infection. *American Journal of Gastroenterology*, 112(2), 212-239.

15. Bharucha, A. E., Dorn, S. D., Lembo, A., & Pressman, A. (2013). American Gastroenterological Association medical position statement on constipation. *Gastroenterology*, 144(1), 211-217.

16. Ford, A. C., Moayyedi, P., Lacy, B. E., Lembo, A. J., Saito, Y. A., Schiller, L. R., ... & Task Force on the Management of Functional Bowel Disorders. (2014). American College of Gastroenterology monograph on the management of irritable bowel syndrome and chronic idiopathic constipation. *American Journal of Gastroenterology*, 109, S2-S26.

17. Katz, P. O., Gerson, L. B., & Vela, M. F. (2013). Guidelines for the diagnosis and management of gastroesophageal reflux disease. *American Journal of Gastroenterology*, 108(3), 308-328.

18. Richter, J. E., & Rubenstein, J. H. (2018). Presentation and epidemiology of gastroesophageal reflux disease. *Gastroenterology*, 154(2), 267-276.

19. American Diabetes Association. (2023). Standards of medical care in diabetes—2023. *Diabetes Care*, 46(Supplement_1), S1-S291.

20. ElSayed, N. A., Aleppo, G., Aroda, V. R., Bannuru, R. R., Brown, F. M., Bruemmer, D., ... & Garg, R. (2023). Glycemic targets: Standards of care in diabetes—2023. *Diabetes Care*, 46(Supplement_1), S97-S110.

21. Jonklaas, J., Bianco, A. C., Bauer, A. J., Burman, K. D., Cappola, A. R., Celi, F. S., ... & Sawka, A. M. (2014). Guidelines for the treatment of hypothyroidism: Prepared by the American Thyroid Association task force on thyroid hormone replacement. *Thyroid*, 24(12), 1670-1751.

22. Garber, J. R., Cobin, R. H., Gharib, H., Hennessey, J. V., Klein, I., Mechanick, J. I., ... & Woeber, K. A. (2012). Clinical practice guidelines for hypothyroidism in adults: Cosponsored by the American Association of Clinical Endocrinologists and the American Thyroid Association. *Thyroid*, 22(12), 1200-1235.

23. American Diabetes Association. (2023). Microvascular complications and foot care: Standards of care in diabetes—2023. *Diabetes Care*, 46(Supplement_1), S203-S215.

24. Singh, N., Armstrong, D. G., & Lipsky, B. A. (2005). Preventing foot ulcers in patients with diabetes. *JAMA*, 293(2), 217-228.

25. Panel on Prevention of Falls in Older Persons, American Geriatrics Society and British Geriatrics Society. (2011). Summary of the updated American Geriatrics Society/British Geriatrics Society clinical practice guideline for prevention of falls in older persons. *Journal of the American Geriatrics Society*, 59(1), 148-157.

26. Morse, J. M. (2009). Preventing patient falls: Establishing a fall intervention program. Springer Publishing Company.

27. National Pressure Injury Advisory Panel. (2019). *Prevention and treatment of pressure ulcers/injuries: Quick reference guide*. Cambridge Media.

28. Braden, B., & Maklebust, J. (2005). Preventing pressure ulcers with the Braden Scale: An update on this easy-to-use tool that

assesses a patient's risk. *American Journal of Nursing*, 105(6), 70-72.

29. Chou, R., Fanciullo, G. J., Fine, P. G., Adler, J. A., Ballantyne, J. C., Davies, P., ... & Miaskowski, C. (2009). Clinical guidelines for the use of chronic opioid therapy in chronic noncancer pain. *The Journal of Pain*, 10(2), 113-130.

30. Institute for Safe Medication Practices. (2018). *ISMP's list of high-alert medications in acute care settings*. Retrieved from https://www.ismp.org/recommendations/high-alert-medications-acute-list

31. The Joint Commission. (2019). *National Patient Safety Goals effective January 2019*. The Joint Commission.

32. Hughes, R. G., & Blegen, M. A. (2008). Medication administration safety. In R. G. Hughes (Ed.), *Patient safety and quality: An evidence-based handbook for nurses* (Chapter 37). Agency for Healthcare Research and Quality.

33. O'Gara, P. T., Kushner, F. G., Ascheim, D. D., Casey Jr, D. E., Chung, M. K., De Lemos, J. A., ... & Zhao, D. X. (2013). 2013 ACCF/AHA guideline for the management of ST-elevation myocardial infarction: A report of the American College of Cardiology Foundation/American Heart Association Task Force on Practice Guidelines. *Journal of the American College of Cardiology*, 61(4), e78-e140.

34. Ibanez, B., James, S., Agewall, S., Antunes, M. J., Bucciarelli-Ducci, C., Bueno, H., ... & Widimský, P. (2018). 2017 ESC Guidelines for the management of acute myocardial infarction in patients presenting with ST-segment elevation. *European Heart Journal*, 39(2), 119-177.

35. Mehta, L. S., Beckie, T. M., DeVon, H. A., Grines, C. L., Krumholz, H. M., Johnson, M. N., ... & Wenger, N. K. (2016). Acute myocardial infarction in women: A scientific statement from the American Heart Association. *Circulation*, 133(9), 916-947.

36. Yancy, C. W., Jessup, M., Bozkurt, B., Butler, J., Casey Jr, D. E., Colvin, M. M., ... & Westlake, C. (2017). 2017 ACC/AHA/HFSA focused update of the 2013 ACCF/AHA guideline for the management of heart failure: A report of the American College of Cardiology/American Heart Association Task Force on Clinical Practice Guidelines. *Journal of the American College of Cardiology*, 70(6), 776-803.

37. Mullens, W., Damman, K., Harjola, V. P., Mebazaa, A., Brunner-La Rocca, H. P., Martens, P., ... & Filippatos, G. (2019). The use of diuretics in heart failure with congestion—a position statement from the Heart Failure Association of the European Society of Cardiology. *European Journal of Heart Failure*, 21(2), 137-155.

38. January, C. T., Wann, L. S., Calkins, H., Chen, L. Y., Cigarroa, J. E., Cleveland Jr, J. C., ... & Yancy, C. W. (2019). 2019 AHA/ACC/HRS focused update of the 2014 AHA/ACC/HRS guideline for the management of patients with atrial fibrillation: A report of the American College of Cardiology/American Heart Association Task Force on Clinical Practice Guidelines. *Journal of the American College of Cardiology*, 74(1), 104-132.

39. Lip, G. Y., Banerjee, A., Boriani, G., Chiang, C. E., Fargo, R., Freedman, B., ... & Zaghloul, A. (2018). Antithrombotic therapy for atrial fibrillation: CHEST guideline and expert panel report. *Chest*, 154(5), 1121-1201.

40. Whelton, P. K., Carey, R. M., Aronow, W. S., Casey Jr, D. E., Collins, K. J., Himmelfarb, C. D., ... & Wright Jr, J. T. (2018). 2017 ACC/AHA/AAPA/ABC/ACPM/AGS/APhA/ASH/ASPC/NMA/PCN A guideline for the prevention, detection, evaluation, and management of high blood pressure in adults: A report of the American College of Cardiology/American Heart Association Task Force on Clinical Practice Guidelines. *Journal of the American College of Cardiology*, 71(19), e127-e248.

41. van den Born, B. J. H., Lip, G. Y., Brguljan-Hitij, J., Cremer, A., Segura, J., Morales, E., ... & Januszewicz, A. (2017). ESC/ESH Guidelines for the management of arterial hypertension: The Task Force for the management of arterial hypertension of the European Society of Cardiology (ESC) and the European Society of Hypertension (ESH). *European Heart Journal*, 38(35), 2629-2630.

42. Global Initiative for Chronic Obstructive Lung Disease. (2023). *Global strategy for the diagnosis, management, and prevention of chronic obstructive pulmonary disease*. GOLD.

43. Rochwerg, B., Brochard, L., Elliott, M. W., Hess, D., Hill, N. S., Nava, S., ... & Raoof, S. (2017). Official ERS/ATS clinical practice guidelines: Noninvasive ventilation for acute respiratory failure. *European Respiratory Journal*, 50(2), 1602426.

44. Osadnik, C. R., Tee, V. S., Carson-Chahhoud, K. V., Picot, J., Wedzicha, J. A., & Smith, B. J. (2017). Non-invasive ventilation for the management of acute hypercapnic respiratory failure due to exacerbation of chronic obstructive pulmonary disease. *Cochrane Database of Systematic Reviews*, (7).

45. Rhodes, A., Evans, L. E., Alhazzani, W., Levy, M. M., Antonelli, M., Ferrer, R., ... & Dellinger, R. P. (2017). Surviving sepsis campaign: International guidelines for management of sepsis and septic shock: 2016. *Intensive Care Medicine*, 43(3), 304-377.

46. Singer, M., Deutschman, C. S., Seymour, C. W., Shankar-Hari, M., Annane, D., Bauer, M., ... & Angus, D. C. (2016). The third international consensus definitions for sepsis and septic shock (Sepsis-3). *JAMA*, 315(8), 801-810.

47. Yang, C. K., Teng, A., Lee, D. Y., & Rose, K. (2017). Pulmonary complications after major abdominal surgery: National Surgical Quality Improvement Program analysis. *Journal of Surgical Research*, 198(2), 441-449.

48. Canet, J., Gallart, L., Gomar, C., Paluzie, G., Vallès, J., Castillo, J., ... & Mazo, V. (2010). Prediction of postoperative pulmonary complications in a population-based surgical cohort. *Anesthesiology*, 113(6), 1338-1350.

49. Kitabchi, A. E., Umpierrez, G. E., Miles, J. M., & Fisher, J. N. (2009). Hyperglycemic crises in adult patients with diabetes. *Diabetes Care*, 32(7), 1335-1343.

50. Wolfsdorf, J. I., Glaser, N., Agus, M., Fritsch, M., Hanas, R., Rewers, A., ... & Codner, E. (2018). ISPAD clinical practice consensus guidelines 2018: Diabetic ketoacidosis and the hyperglycemic hyperosmolar state. *Pediatric Diabetes*, 19, 155-177.

51. Dhatariya, K. K., Glaser, N. S., Codner, E., & Umpierrez, G. E. (2020). Diabetic ketoacidosis. *Nature Reviews Disease Primers*, 6(1), 1-20.

52. Joint British Diabetes Societies Inpatient Care Group. (2013). *The management of diabetic ketoacidosis in adults*. NHS Diabetes.

53. Laine, L., & Jensen, D. M. (2012). Management of patients with ulcer bleeding. *American Journal of Gastroenterology*, 107(3), 345-360.

54. Mehta, R. L., Kellum, J. A., Shah, S. V., Molitoris, B. A., Ronco, C., Warnock, D. G., & Levin, A. (2007). Acute Kidney Injury Network: Report of an initiative to improve outcomes in acute kidney injury. *Critical Care*, 11(2), 1-8.

55. Khwaja, A. (2012). KDIGO clinical practice guidelines for acute kidney injury. *Nephron Clinical Practice*, 120(4), c179-c184.

56. Powers, W. J., Rabinstein, A. A., Ackerson, T., Adeoye, O. M., Bambakidis, N. C., Becker, K., ... & Tirschwell, D. L. (2019). Guidelines for the early management of patients with acute ischemic stroke: 2019 update to the 2018 guidelines for the

early management of acute ischemic stroke. *Stroke*, 50(12), e344-e418.

57. Martino, R., Foley, N., Bhogal, S., Diamant, N., Speechley, M., & Teasell, R. (2005). Dysphagia after stroke: Incidence, diagnosis, and pulmonary complications. *Stroke*, 36(12), 2756-2763.

58. van Diepen, S., Katz, J. N., Albert, N. M., Henry, T. D., Jacobs, A. K., Kapur, N. K., ... & Thiele, H. (2017). Contemporary management of cardiogenic shock: A scientific statement from the American Heart Association. *Circulation*, 136(16), e232-e268.

59. Thiele, H., Ohman, E. M., de Waha-Thiele, S., Zeymer, U., & Desch, S. (2019). Management of cardiogenic shock complicating myocardial infarction: An update 2019. *European Heart Journal*, 40(32), 2671-2683.

60. Panchal, A. R., Bartos, J. A., Cabañas, J. G., Donnino, M. W., Drennan, I. R., Hirsch, K. G., ... & Magid, D. J. (2020). Part 3: Adult basic and advanced life support: 2020 American Heart Association guidelines for cardiopulmonary resuscitation and emergency cardiovascular care. *Circulation*, 142(16_suppl_2), S366-S468.

61. Neumar, R. W., Shuster, M., Callaway, C. W., Gent, L. M., Atkins, D. L., Bhanji, F., ... & Hazinski, M. F. (2015). Part 1: Executive summary: 2015 American Heart Association guidelines update for cardiopulmonary resuscitation and emergency cardiovascular care. *Circulation*, 132(18_suppl_2), S315-S367.

62. Holcomb, J. B., Tilley, B. C., Baraniuk, S., Fox, E. E., Wade, C. E., Podbielski, J. M., ... & Schreiber, M. A. (2015). Transfusion of plasma, platelets, and red blood cells in a 1:1:1 vs a 1:1:2 ratio and mortality in patients with severe trauma: The PROPPR randomized clinical trial. *JAMA*, 313(5), 471-482.

63. Institute of Medicine. (2015). *Dying in America: Improving quality and honoring individual preferences near the end of life*. National Academies Press.

64. Holbrook, A., Schulman, S., Witt, D. M., Vandvik, P. O., Fish, J., Kovacs, M. J., ... & Guyatt, G. H. (2012). Evidence-based management of anticoagulant therapy: Antithrombotic Therapy and Prevention of Thrombosis, 9th ed: American College of Chest Physicians Evidence-Based Clinical Practice Guidelines. *Chest*, 141(2_suppl), e152S-e184S.

65. Ageno, W., Gallus, A. S., Wittkowsky, A., Crowther, M., Hylek, E. M., & Palareti, G. (2012). Oral anticoagulant therapy: Antithrombotic Therapy and Prevention of Thrombosis, 9th ed: American College of Chest Physicians Evidence-Based Clinical Practice Guidelines. *Chest*, 141(2_suppl), e44S-e88S.

66. By the 2019 American Geriatrics Society Beers Criteria® Update Expert Panel. (2019). American Geriatrics Society 2019 updated AGS Beers Criteria® for potentially inappropriate medication use in older adults. *Journal of the American Geriatrics Society*, 67(4), 674-694.

67. American Diabetes Association. (2023). Glycemic targets: Standards of care in diabetes—2023. *Diabetes Care*, 46(Supplement_1), S97-S110.

68. Yawn, B. P., Buchanan, G. R., Afenyi-Annan, A. N., Ballas, S. K., Hassell, K. L., James, A. H., ... & John-Sowah, J. (2014). Management of sickle cell disease: summary of the 2014 evidence-based report by expert panel members. *JAMA*, 312(10), 1033-1048.

69. Brandow, A. M., Carroll, C. P., Creary, S., Edwards-Elliott, R., Glassberg, J., Hurley, R. W., ... & Smith, W. R. (2020). American Society of Hematology 2020 guidelines for sickle cell disease: management of acute and chronic pain. *Blood Advances*, 4(12), 2656-2701.

70. Rhodes, A., Evans, L. E., Alhazzani, W., Levy, M. M., Antonelli, M., Ferrer, R., ... & Dellinger, R. P. (2017). Surviving sepsis campaign: International guidelines for management of sepsis and septic shock: 2016. *Intensive Care Medicine*, 43(3), 304-377.

71. Fan, E., Brodie, D., & Slutsky, A. S. (2018). Acute respiratory distress syndrome: Advances in diagnosis and treatment. *JAMA*, 319(7), 698-710.

72. Jenkins, J. L., McCarthy, M. L., Sauer, L. M., Green, G. B., Stuart, S., Thomas, T. L., & Hsu, E. B. (2008). Mass-casualty triage: Time for an evidence-based approach. *Prehospital and Disaster Medicine*, 23(1), 3-8.

73. Smith, G. B., Prytherch, D. R., Meredith, P., Schmidt, P. E., & Featherstone, P. I. (2013). The ability of the National Early Warning Score (NEWS) to discriminate patients at risk of early cardiac arrest, unanticipated intensive care unit admission, and death. *Resuscitation*, 84(4), 465-470.

74. Petersen, J. A., Antonsen, K., & Rasmussen, L. S. (2016). Frequency of early warning score assessment and clinical deterioration in hospitalized patients: A randomized trial. *Resuscitation*, 101, 91-96.

75. Amsterdam, E. A., Wenger, N. K., Brindis, R. G., Casey Jr, D. E., Ganiats, T. G., Holmes Jr, D. R., ... & Zieman, S. J. (2014). 2014 AHA/ACC guideline for the management of patients with non-ST-elevation acute coronary syndromes: A report of the American College of Cardiology/American Heart Association Task Force on Practice Guidelines. *Journal of the American College of Cardiology*, 64(24), e139-e228.

76. Collet, J. P., Thiele, H., Barbato, E., Barthélémy, O., Bauersachs, J., Bhatt, D. L., ... & Siontis, G. C. (2021). 2020 ESC Guidelines for the management of acute coronary syndromes in patients presenting without persistent ST-segment elevation. *European Heart Journal*, 42(14), 1289-1367.

77. Hillis, L. D., Smith, P. K., Anderson, J. L., Bittl, J. A., Bridges, C. R., Byrne, J. G., ... & Winniford, M. D. (2011). 2011 ACCF/AHA guideline for coronary artery bypass graft surgery: A report of the American College of Cardiology Foundation/American Heart Association Task Force on Practice Guidelines. *Circulation*, 124(23), e652-e735.

78. Adler, Y., Charron, P., Imazio, M., Badano, L., Barón-Esquivias, G., Bogaert, J., ... & Zamorano, J. L. (2015). 2015 ESC Guidelines for the diagnosis and management of pericardial diseases: The Task Force for the Diagnosis and Management of Pericardial Diseases of the European Society of Cardiology (ESC). *European Heart Journal*, 36(42), 2921-2964.

79. Ginès, P., Guevara, M., Arroyo, V., & Rodés, J. (2003). Hepatorenal syndrome. *The Lancet*, 362(9398), 1819-1827.

80. Salerno, F., Gerbes, A., Ginès, P., Wong, F., & Arroyo, V. (2007). Diagnosis, prevention and treatment of hepatorenal syndrome in cirrhosis. *Gut*, 56(9), 1310-1318.

81. Banks, P. A., Bollen, T. L., Dervenis, C., Gooszen, H. G., Johnson, C. D., Sarr, M. G., ... & Vege, S. S. (2013). Classification of acute pancreatitis—2012: revision of the Atlanta classification and definitions by international consensus. *Gut*, 62(1), 102-111.

82. Tenner, S., Baillie, J., DeWitt, J., & Vege, S. S. (2013). American College of Gastroenterology guideline: management of acute pancreatitis. *American Journal of Gastroenterology*, 108(9), 1400-1415.

83. Yadav, D., O'Connell, M., & Papachristou, G. I. (2013). Natural history following the first attack of acute pancreatitis. *American Journal of Gastroenterology*, 108(9), 1467-1475.

84. van Santvoort, H. C., Besselink, M. G., Bakker, O. J., Hofker, H. S., Boermeester, M. A., Dejong, C. H., ... & Gooszen, H. G. (2010). A step-up approach or open necrosectomy for

necrotizing pancreatitis. *New England Journal of Medicine*, 362(16), 1491-1502.

85. Beauchamp, T. L., & Childress, J. F. (2019). *Principles of biomedical ethics* (8th ed.). Oxford University Press.

86. Appelbaum, P. S. (2007). Assessment of patients' competence to consent to treatment. *New England Journal of Medicine*, 357(18), 1834-1840.

87. Umscheid, C. A., Mitchell, M. D., Doshi, J. A., Agarwal, R., Williams, K., & Brennan, P. J. (2011). Estimating the proportion of healthcare-associated infections that are reasonably preventable and the related mortality and costs. *Infection Control & Hospital Epidemiology*, 32(2), 101-114.

88. Coleman, E. A., Parry, C., Chalmers, S., & Min, S. J. (2006). The care transitions intervention: results of a randomized controlled trial. *Archives of Internal Medicine*, 166(17), 1822-1828.

www.ingramcontent.com/pod-product-compliance
Lightning Source LLC
Chambersburg PA
CBHW070812270326
41927CB00010B/2384